WILLIAMS-SONOMA
COLLECTION

HEALTHY MAIN DISHES

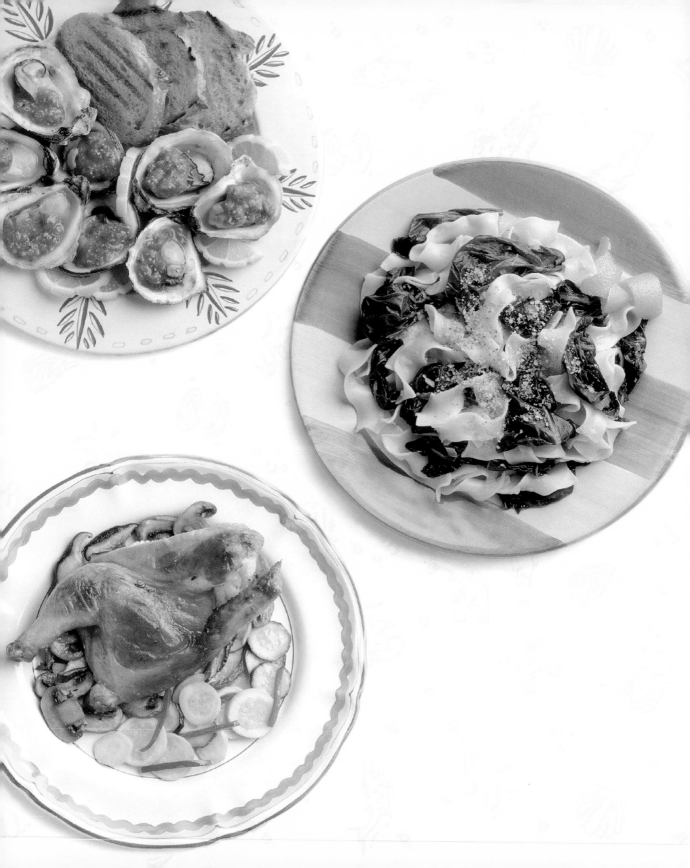

WILLIAMS-SONOMA
COLLECTION

HEALTHY
MAIN
DISHES

GENERAL EDITOR

CHUCK WILLIAMS

RECIPES BY

CYNTHIA HIZER

PHOTOGRAPHY BY

ALLAN ROSENBERG & ALLEN V. LOTT

TIME
LIFE
BOOKS

**Time-Life Books is a division of
Time-Life Incorporated**

President & CEO: John Fahey, Jr.

TIME-LIFE BOOKS

President, Time-Life Books: John D. Hall
Vice President & Publisher: Terry Newell
Director of New Product Development: Regina Hall
Director of Financial Operations: J. Brian Birky
Editorial Director: Donia Ann Steele

WILLIAMS-SONOMA
Founder: Chuck Williams

WELDON OWEN INC.
President: John Owen
Publisher/Vice President: Wendely Harvey
Associate Publisher: Tori Ritchie
Project Coordinator: Jill Fox
Consulting Editor: Norman Kolpas
Recipe Analysis & Nutritional Consultation:
    Hill Nutrition Associates Inc.
    Lynne S. Hill, MS, RD; William A. Hill, MS, RD
Copy Editor: Sharon Silva
Art Director: John Bull
Designer: Patty Hill
Production Director: Stephanie Sherman
Production Editor: Janique Gascoigne
Co-Editions Director: Derek Barton
Co-Editions Production Manager: Tarji Mickelson
Food & Prop Stylist: Heidi Gintner
Associate Food & Prop Stylist: Danielle Di Salvo
Assistant Food Stylists: Michelle Syracuse, Nette Scott
Props Courtesy: Sandra Griswold
Indexer: ALTA Indexing Service
Proofreaders: Ken DellaPenta, Desne Border
Illustrator: Diana Reiss-Koncar
Special Thanks: Claire Sanchez, Marguerite Ozburn,
    Jennifer Mullins, Mick Bagnato

The Williams-Sonoma Healthy Collection
conceived & produced by Weldon Owen Inc.
814 Montgomery Street, San Francisco, CA 94133

In collaboration with Williams-Sonoma
3250 Van Ness Avenue, San Francisco, CA 94109

Production by Mandarin Offset, Hong Kong
Printed in China

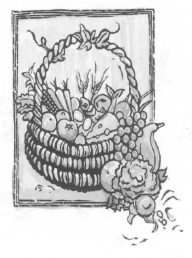

A Weldon Owen Production

Library of Congress
Cataloging-in-Publication Data:

Hizer, Cynthia.
    Healthy main dishes / general editor, Chuck Williams ;
recipes by Cynthia Hizer ; photography by Allan Rosenberg
& Allen V. Lott.
        p.   cm. — (Williams-Sonoma collection)
    Includes index.
    ISBN 0-7835-4600-9
    1. Entrées (Cookery)   2. Nutrition.   I. Williams, Chuck.
II. Title.   III. Series.
TX740.H577   1995
641.8'2—dc20   95-10207
                                    CIP

*Cover: Turkey fillets (recipe on page 16) expand the use of this
lowfat meat from its special occasion status. Back Cover: Colorful
Lemon-Black Pepper Pasta (recipe on page 85) makes a quick
main dish or light one-dish meal.*

HEALTHY
MAIN
DISHES

CONTENTS

THE BASICS

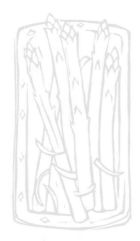

$\mathcal{T}$he aim of the main dish recipes and nutritional information on these pages is to help you in your quest to eat a balanced diet without giving up culinary pleasures. While in no way a weight-loss guide, this book offers a wealth of information, inspiration and recipes tailored to a healthier way of eating. A consensus of experts considers a healthy diet one in which 30 percent or fewer calories come from fat, about 15 percent from protein and about 55 percent from complex carbohydrates, and that is high in fiber and low in cholesterol and added salt. More than that, a healthy diet is one that uses a variety of fresh foods, cooked in interesting ways that are enjoyable to eat. This chapter begins where a healthy diet begins, with guidelines for choosing the best ingredients, including tips on purchasing and storing food for greatest flavor. It ends with definitions of the nutrient information listed for each recipe in *Healthy Main Dishes*.

COOKING HEALTHY MAIN DISHES

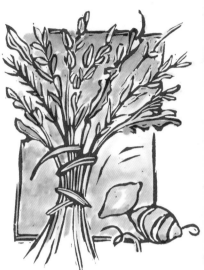

By keeping in mind just a few basic principles, you can start immediately to cook healthier main dishes that contribute to a nutritionally balanced diet—one that is widely varied in nutrients, offers adequate protein, and is higher in complex carbohydrates and fiber and lower in fat and cholesterol.

The secret to success lies not in any radical changes so much as in subtly altering the way you already shop, cook and eat. Begin by making healthy choices when you shop for main dish ingredients using the information on these pages as a guide.

Then, let the recipes in this book inspire you to cook a varied diet that provides a full range of nutrients. As you look through and try these main dishes, note the many ways in which they add bright, appealing flavor without the use of excessive fat, cholesterol or salt. Such ingredients as herbs, spices, vinegars, wine and citrus fruits enliven your cooking in fresh, healthy new ways.

Finally, serve and eat portions that emphasize vegetables, pastas, grains and rice over meat, poultry and seafood. In no time at all, you'll be on your way to a healthier diet.

CUTTING THE FAT

More than any other change you make in the way you eat, reducing the amount of fat you consume will help you achieve a healthier diet. The following tips can help you reduce the fat in your diet.

CHOOSE LOWFAT COOKING METHODS

Use cooking methods that require little or no added fat—broiling, roasting, braising—instead of frying.

COOK WITH LESS OIL

Just a thin film of oil in a pan is sufficient to brown foods. When possible, use nonstick pans, nonstick cooking sprays or no oil at all.

REDUCE PORTIONS OF ANIMAL PROTEIN

Limit portions of cooked lean meat, poultry or fish to 3 ounces—about the size of a deck of cards.

MAKE LEAN CHOICES

Shop for cuts of meat that are naturally lower in fat, saturated fat and cholesterol (see page 10).

STRIP OFF SKIN

When cooking poultry, remove the skin before cooking if the recipe allows; or, if the poultry is cooked with its skin on, pull off the skin before eating.

TRIM OFF VISIBLE FAT

Before cooking, cut or pull off all visible fat from the surface of meat or poultry.

MAKE THE RIGHT FAT CHOICES

Instead of cooking with butter or other animal fat, use an unsaturated vegetable oil that does not increase blood cholesterol levels. Monounsaturated oils such as olive, canola or peanut oil have been found actually to help lower blood cholesterol.

POUR, SKIM OR SCRAPE OFF EXCESS FAT

After browning meat, pour off any fat from the pan. When braising or otherwise simmering meat, poultry or seafood, drape a paper towel across the surface and pull it away to soak up the fat. When a stew, stock or other cooking liquid has cooled, spoon or scrape off any fat congealed on the surface.

MAKING HEALTHY CHOICES

The choices you make when shopping directly affect the bottom line of your daily and weekly nutritional intake. Use the following basic information on featured main dish ingredients—poultry, meats, complex carbohydrates and seafood—as a guide to making healthy choices.

CHOOSING POULTRY

Your healthiest choice for poultry main dishes is unquestionably the skinless breast meat of chicken or turkey, which has far less fat than a comparable skinless portion of dark meat (see chart). That doesn't mean, however, that you should avoid dark meat; cooked skinless and with little or no added fat, and combined with other lowfat or fat-free ingredients, it still contributes to a healthy diet.

POULTRY TYPE

3 OZ/90 G COOKED	CALORIES	FAT (G)	SATURATED FAT (G)	CHOLESTEROL (MG)
Chicken breast, skinless	141	3.0	0.7	72
Chicken thigh, skinless	178	9.2	2.1	80
Turkey light meat, skinless	133	2.7	0.7	59
Turkey dark meat, skinless	159	6.1	1.8	73

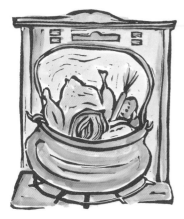

Seek out the best-quality poultry in your area by asking around to find the best butchers or poulterers. Ask them about the source of their poultry. So-called free-range birds, which can hunt and peck for more varied diets, usually are more flavorful, but factory-raised poultry that was provided with a good diet of grains can also taste good.

When buying any poultry, the signs of freshness to look for include creamy yellow or creamy white skin that looks moist and supple, with well-distributed yellow fat; avoid any chicken, with or without skin, that looks dried out, discolored, blemished or bruised. Any "off" smells indicate that the poultry is less than fresh. Check the "sell by" date on prepackaged poultry. At home, store poultry in the coldest part of the refrigerator, with its wrappings loosened, and cook within 2 days of purchase. Always wash and pat dry poultry prior to cooking.

CHOOSING MEAT

Though higher in calories, fat and cholesterol than most comparably sized portions of poultry or seafood, meat still can play a significant role in a healthy diet, contributing complete protein, iron and many other essential nutrients. The key to eating meat is to make your main dish selections from among the leanest cuts, such as chuck, round, loin or leg, which generally come from larger, more active muscles (see chart, which lists values for cuts used in this book); to cook them in ways that minimize fat; and to limit cooked portions to no more than 3 ounces/90 grams (5 ounces/ 155 grams raw), extending the meat by combining it with vegetables and complex carbohydrates such as rice, beans, pasta, potatoes and grains.

CUT OF MEAT

3 oz/90 g Cooked, trimmed	Calories	Fat (g)	Saturated Fat (g)	Cholesterol (mg)
Beef flank steak	176	8.6	3.7	57
Tenderloin	179	8.5	3.2	71
Lean ground beef	231	15.7	6.2	74
Lamb loin	183	8.3	3.0	80
Pork center loin	165	6.1	2.2	66
Pork tenderloin	133	4.1	1.6	67

When shopping for meat, avoid prime cuts, which are usually highest in fat. Look for beef or lamb that is bright red in color, and pork that is a clear, pale pink. Vacuum-packaged meat may appear purplish, but will brighten in color on exposure to air. Excess fat should be trimmed from the meat. At home, store the meat in the coldest part of your refrigerator, with its wrappings loosened; cook whole cuts within 3 to 4 days, ground meat within 1 to 2 days.

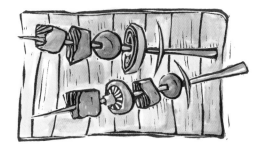

CHOOSING PASTAS, GRAINS & BEANS

In recent years, grains (including grain pastas) and legumes (beans, peas and lentils) have gained favor as health-conscious cooks realize these inexpensive ingredients yield satisfying main dishes that are high in protein and dietary fiber and low in fat. And, like all plant foods, grains and legumes contain no cholesterol.

Unlike all animal proteins, however, no single plant source contains all nine of the essential amino acids that are necessary for good nutrition. For that reason, these ingredients should be eaten in complementary combinations—such as the classic pairing of rice and beans—to form complete proteins.

Grains are the seed kernels of cereal plants. Some are processed after harvesting to make them easier to cook. Usually, the more processing done, the more fiber, vitamins and proteins lost. Choosing whole grains over polished grains adds significantly to the nutrients derived from grains.

Store pastas, grains and beans in tightly covered containers away from light.

CHOOSING FISH & SHELLFISH

Seafood offers today's cook some of the healthiest options for main dish animal protein, being lower in overall fat than meat or poultry while containing the same general levels of cholesterol and low saturated fat. In addition, many fish species—particularly fattier varieties such as salmon, tuna, mackerel and sardines—contain a healthy bonus: omega-3 fatty acids, which some medical studies have found to play a role in preventing heart disease.

When shopping for fish, seek out the most reputable seafood shop in your area, with varied selections and a frequent turnover of product. The freshest seafood has a clean, fresh scent of the ocean, so avoid anything that smells fishy. Fish fillets or steaks should look moist, bright and lustrous, with no discoloration or drying. Whole fish should have bright, shiny, well-attached scales; bright pink or red gills; bright, clear eyes and firm, elastic flesh that is springy to the touch.

Shellfish should also smell absolutely fresh and should be alive when purchased; avoid or discard any specimens with shells that gape open and do not close tightly when handled.

Whenever possible, purchase fresh rather than frozen fish. If the fish has been frozen, buy it frozen, not defrosted, and defrost it in the refrigerator at home just prior to cooking. Never refreeze thawed fish. Store fresh fish dry, in one layer in a baking dish lined with paper and covered with plastic wrap in the refrigerator and use within 24 hours of purchase.

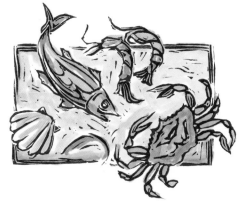

Refrigerate shellfish as soon as possible after purchase. For best results, store shellfish on a bed of ice in the refrigerator or an ice chest covered with a damp towel. Use within a few days.

FISH SUBSTITUTES

Fish that are similar in size, texture, taste and fat content can usually be used interchangeably in recipes.

LEAN–DELICATE
(Contains less than 2.5 percent fat)
Small flounders, including plaice, gray sole, winter flounder and yellowtail; soles including English, petrale, rex and sand dab

LEAN–DENSE
Halibut; large grouper including giant, Nassau and Warsaw; bluenose; shark

LEAN–MEDIUM-DENSE
Freshwater bass; cods including Antarctic queen, Atlantic whiting, haddock, hake, hoki and pollack; large flounders including arrowtooth, southern and summer; halibut; John Dory; kingklip; lingcod; perch including walleye and yellow; northern pike; rockfish including ocean perch; Pacific snapper and red snapper

MODERATELY LEAN–DENSE
(Contains less than 5 percent fat)
Cobia; mackerel; moonfish; sturgeon; swordfish; tuna

MODERATELY LEAN–MEDIUM-DENSE
Freshwater catfish; grouper; mahi mahi; salmon including chum and pink papio; rainbow trout; sea bass; sea bream including porgy, scup and sheepshead; seatrout; snook; tautog

OILIER–MILD FLAVORED
(Contains more than 5 percent fat)
Freshwater buffalo; freshwater carp; Greenland turbot; orange roughy; sablefish including black cod and butterfish; lake trout; lake whitefish

OILIER–DISTINCT FLAVOR
Barracuda; herring; mackerel; mullet; pompano and salmon including Atlantic, king (chinook) and silver (coho)

CHOOSING HERBS

Many fresh and dried herbs enhance the flavor of healthy main dishes without adding fat, calories or sodium. In general, fresh herbs are added towards the end of cooking, as their flavor dissipates with long exposure to heat; dried herbs may be used in dishes that cook longer, and measure for measure are generally twice as concentrated in flavor as their fresh counterparts.

BASIL
A sweet, spicy herb popular in Italian and French dishes. The flavor of fresh basil is far more powerful than and superior to dried basil.

BAY LEAVES
Dried whole leaves of the bay laurel tree are pungent and spicy. They flavor simmered dishes, marinades and pickling mixtures. Because the edges can be sharp, always remove and discard leaves before serving.

CHIVES
Both the long, thin green shoot and purple flower are edible, with a mild flavor reminiscent of the onion, to which it is related. Add them to potato dishes. Garlic chives have a similarly mild flavor that is reminiscent of garlic.

CILANTRO
This green, leafy herb resembling flat-leaf (Italian) parsley, with a sharp, aromatic, somewhat astringent flavor, is popular in Latin American and Asian cuisines. It is sometimes called fresh coriander or Chinese parsley. The seeds of the same plant are called coriander.

DILL
These fine, feathery leaves with a sweet, aromatic flavor are sold fresh or dried. Try them with egg dishes.

MINT
A refreshing herb available in many varieties, with spearmint the most common. Used fresh to flavor a broad range of savory and sweet dishes, including lamb and cold chicken dishes.

OREGANO
An aromatic, pungent and spicy Mediterranean herb used fresh or dried as a seasoning for all kinds of savory dishes. Especially popular in tomato and pasta dishes.

PARSLEY
This popular fresh herb is available in two varieties, the readily available curly-leaf type and a flat-leaf type. The latter, also known as Italian parsley, has a more pronounced flavor and is preferred on many types of food.

ROSEMARY
A Mediterranean herb, used either fresh or dried, its aromatic flavor is well suited to lamb, veal, poultry, seafood and vegetables. Strong in flavor, it should be used sparingly, except when grilling.

SAGE
This pungent herb, used either fresh or dried, goes particularly well with fresh or cured pork, lamb, veal or poultry.

TARRAGON
A fragrant, distinctively sweet herb used fresh or dried as a seasoning for salads, seafood, poultry, eggs and vegetables.

THYME
This fragrant, clean-tasting, small-leaved herb is popular fresh or dried as a seasoning for poultry, pork, seafood or vegetables. A variety called lemon thyme imparts a pleasant lemon scent to foods.

READING A NUTRITIONAL CHART

Each recipe in this book has been analyzed for nutritional composition by a registered dietitian. Beside each recipe, a chart similar to the one below lists the nutrient breakdown per serving. Use these numbers as a tool when putting together meals—and weeks and months of meals—designed for a healthy eating style.

All ingredients listed within each recipe have been included in the nutritional analysis. Exceptions are items added "to taste" and those listed as "optional." When seasoning with salt, bear in mind that you are adding 2,200 mg of sodium for each teaspoon of regular salt and 1,800 mg per teaspoon of coarse kosher or sea salt. The addition of black, white or red pepper does not alter nutrient values. Substituted ingredients, recipe variations and side dishes suggested in recipe introductions or shown in photographs have not been included in the analysis.

Quantities are based on a single serving of each recipe.

Protein, one of the basic life-giving nutrients, helps build and repair body tissues and performs other essential functions. One gram of protein contains 4 calories. A healthy diet derives about 15% of daily calories from protein.

Total fat is a measure of the grams of fat present in a serving, with 1 gram of fat equivalent to 9 calories (more than twice the calories in a gram of protein or carbohydrates). Experts recommend that fat intake be limited to a maximum of 30% of total calories.

Cholesterol is present in foods of animal origin. Experts suggest a daily intake of no more than 300 mg. Plant foods contain no cholesterol.

Nutritional Analysis Per Serving:

**CALORIES 211
(KILOJOULES 887)
PROTEIN 42 G
CARBOHYDRATES 0 G
TOTAL FAT 4 G
SATURATED FAT 1 G
CHOLESTEROL 105 MG
SODIUM 84 MG
DIETARY FIBER 0 G**

Calories (Kilojoules) provide a measure of the energy provided by any given food. A calorie equals the heat energy necessary to raise the temperature of 1 kg of water by 1 degree Celsius. One calorie is equal to 4.2 kilojoules—a term used instead of calories in some countries.

Carbohydrates, classed as either simple (sugars) or complex (starches), are the main source of dietary energy. One gram of carbohydrates contains 4 calories. A healthy diet derives about 55% of calories from carbohydrates, with no more than 10% coming from sugars.

Saturated fat, derived from animal products and some tropical oils, has been found to raise blood cholesterol, and should be limited to no more than one third of total fat calories.

Sodium, derived from salt and naturally present in many foods, helps maintain a proper balance of body fluids. Excess intake can lead to high blood pressure or hypertension in sodium-sensitive people. Those not sensitive should limit intake to about 2,400 mg daily.

Fiber in food aids elimination and helps prevent heart disease, intestinal disease and some forms of cancer. A healthy diet should include 20–35 grams of fiber daily.

A Note on Weights and Measures:
All recipes include customary U.S. and metric measurements. Metric conversions are based on a standard developed for these books and have been rounded off. Actual weights may vary. Unless otherwise stated, the recipes were designed for medium-sized fruits and vegetables.

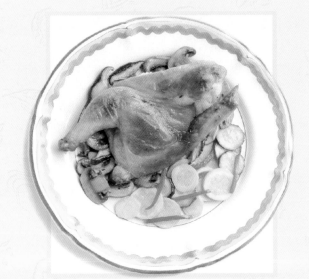

POULTRY & MEAT

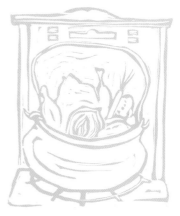

A fiery stew of pork and green chilies; roast lamb chops fragrant with fresh mint; skewers of marinated steak, onions and peppers: Such appetite-stirring images, seen on the following pages, should forever end the notion that healthy eating and red meat are mutually exclusive. Along with the poultry recipes in this chapter, the beef, pork and lamb dishes play a significant role in a healthy diet. The key comes in choosing the leanest cuts of meat or poultry (see pages 9–10), trimming cuts of visible fat, cooking them in ways that minimize added fat, limiting protein portion sizes, extending meals with vegetables and complex carbohydrates and using imaginative seasonings to make every bite more satisfying. Even when a particular preparation is relatively rich, accompany it with a lowfat first course, side dish and dessert for a well-rounded meal in which 30 percent or fewer calories come from fat. See how these simple steps restore meat and poultry to their fitting place on the healthy table.

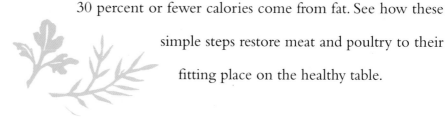

Widely available in food stores, turkey fillets—slices cut from a whole raw turkey breast—make a delicious and satisfying lowfat main dish, served here with golden and red beets.

Turkey Fillets

Serves 6

6 turkey fillets, 6 oz (185 g) each
1 tablespoon olive oil
3 tablespoons balsamic vinegar
1 tablespoon fresh thyme leaves, plus fresh thyme sprigs
1 tablespoon juniper berries, lightly crushed

1. Place the turkey fillets between 2 sheets of plastic wrap and pound gently with the smooth side of a meat mallet until they are ¼ inch (6 mm) thick.

2. Lay the fillets in a single layer in a shallow, nonreactive dish. In a small bowl, stir together the olive oil and balsamic vinegar. Brush the mixture evenly over the fillets. Sprinkle the fillets with the thyme leaves and juniper berries. Cover and refrigerate for 1 hour.

3. Coat a large frying pan with nonstick cooking spray and place over medium-high heat. When the pan is hot, add the fillets, thyme leaves and juniper berries. Cook, turning once, until lightly browned and cooked through, about 2 minutes on each side.

4. To serve, slice the cooked meat and fan the slices onto individual plates. Garnish with thyme sprigs.

Nutritional Analysis
Per Serving:

Calories 211
(Kilojoules 887)
Protein 42 g
Carbohydrates 0 g
Total Fat 4 g
Saturated Fat 1 g
Cholesterol 105 mg
Sodium 84 mg
Dietary Fiber 0 g

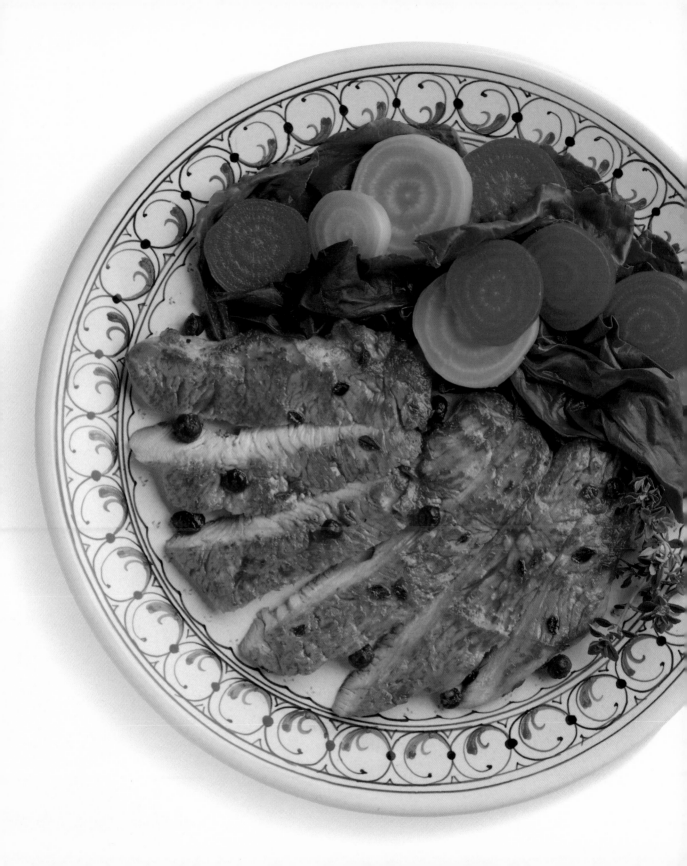

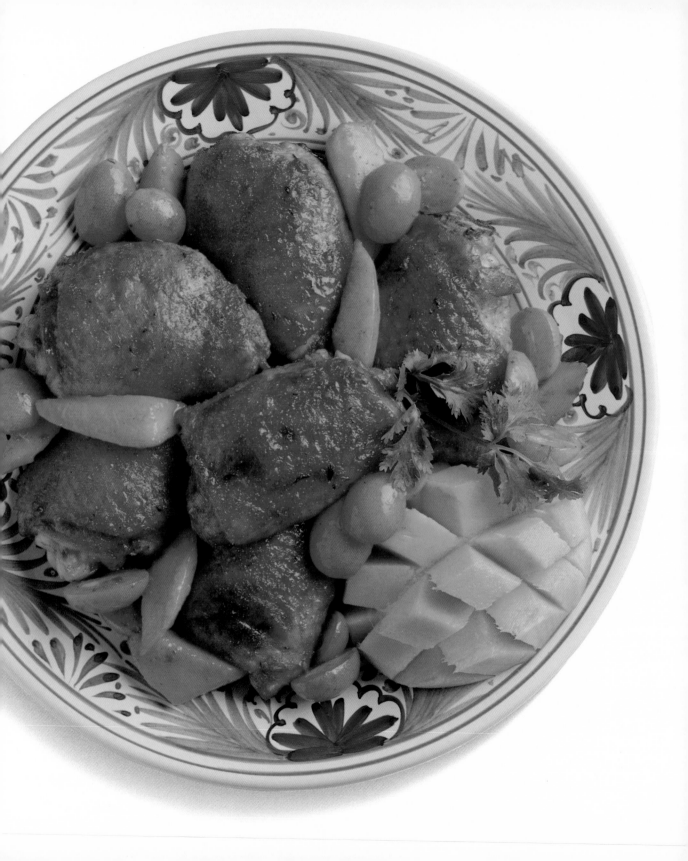

Five-spice powder contributes an exotic accent to roasted chicken thighs. For even more fragrant results, add chunks of mango or whole kumquats to the pan for the last 10 minutes of cooking. Skin the chicken after cooking to cut out more fat.

Seasoned Roast Chicken

Serves 6

6 chicken thighs, 4 oz (125 g) each
1 teaspoon five-spice powder
2 tablespoons brown sugar
2 tablespoons dry sherry

2 tablespoons Roast Garlic Sauce
  (recipe on page 126) or 2 garlic cloves,
  peeled and minced and mixed with
  1 tablespoon white wine vinegar

1. Preheat an oven to 350°F (180°C).
2. Place the chicken thighs in a roasting pan. In a small bowl, stir together the five-spice powder, brown sugar, sherry and Garlic Sauce. Rub the paste evenly over each piece.
3. Roast, basting occasionally with the pan juices, until the juices run clear when the thighs are pierced with a knife and the skin is golden brown and crisp, about 45 minutes.
4. To serve, transfer to a serving platter.

Nutritional Analysis Per Serving:

**CALORIES 176
(KILOJOULES 738)
PROTEIN 15 G
CARBOHYDRATES 6 G
TOTAL FAT 10 G
SATURATED FAT 3 G
CHOLESTEROL 54 MG
SODIUM 52 MG
DIETARY FIBER 0 G**

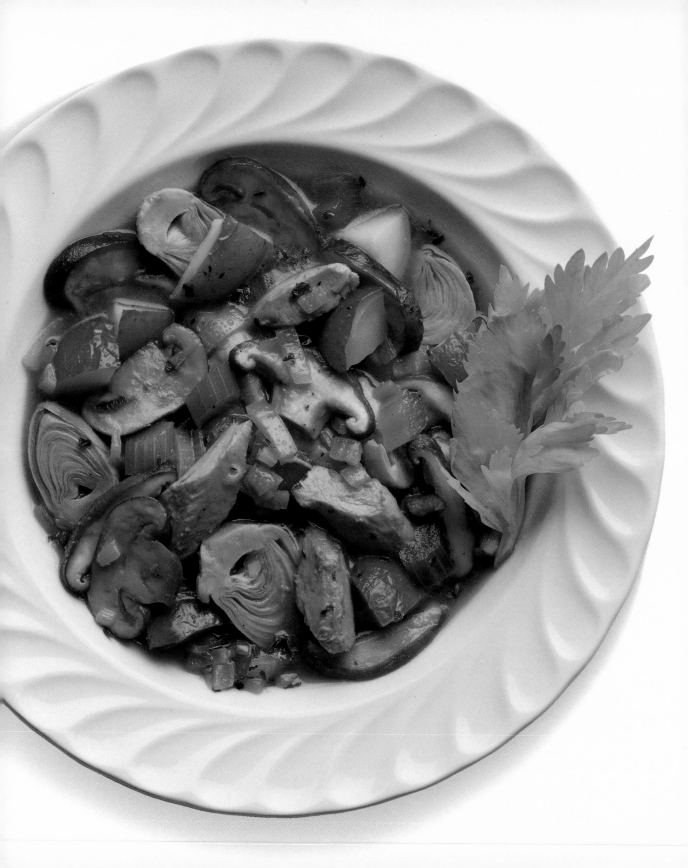

A delicious way to use leftover roast chicken and potatoes, this hearty stew will work well with thawed frozen or drained bottled artichoke hearts. If the robust-flavored shiitake and cremini mushrooms are not available, substitute portobellos or standard button mushrooms.

CHICKEN & ARTICHOKE RAGOUT

Serves 6

2 tablespoons unsalted butter

1 large yellow onion, diced

¼ lb (125 g) fresh shiitake mushrooms, thickly sliced

¼ lb (125 g) fresh cremini mushrooms, thickly sliced

1 celeriac, peeled and diced, or 2 celery stalks with leaves, diced

10 oz (315 g) artichoke hearts

1⅔ cups (10 oz/315 g) skinned cooked chicken meat, cut in 1-inch (2.5-cm) dice

1 cup (5 oz/155 g) diced cooked or roasted potatoes

½ cup (4 fl oz/125 ml) red wine

1 teaspoon fennel seeds

2 tablespoons Roast Garlic Sauce *(recipe on page 126)* or 2 garlic cloves, peeled and minced and mixed with 1 tablespoon white wine vinegar

2 teaspoons herbes de Provence or 1 teaspoon each dried oregano and thyme

8 cups (64 fl oz/2 l) Vegetable Stock or Chicken Stock *(recipes on page 124)* or water

½ teaspoon salt

¼ teaspoon freshly ground pepper

1. In a large saucepan over medium-low heat, melt the butter. Add the onion and sauté until fragrant and translucent, 3–4 minutes. Add the shiitake and cremini mushrooms and continue to sauté, stirring occasionally, until the mushrooms are soft, about 5 minutes.
2. Add the celeriac or celery, artichoke hearts, chicken, potatoes, wine, fennel seeds, Garlic Sauce, herbs, Vegetable or Chicken Stock or water, salt and pepper. Stir to mix well. Bring to a boil, reduce the heat to low, cover and cook until all the ingredients are thoroughly cooked and the flavors have melded, about 30 minutes.
3. To serve, transfer to a large bowl and serve at the table in soup plates or shallow bowls.

Nutritional Analysis Per Serving:

CALORIES 230
(KILOJOULES 964)
PROTEIN 18 G
CARBOHYDRATES 22 G
TOTAL FAT 9 G
SATURATED FAT 3 G
CHOLESTEROL 52 MG
SODIUM 296 MG
DIETARY FIBER 4 G

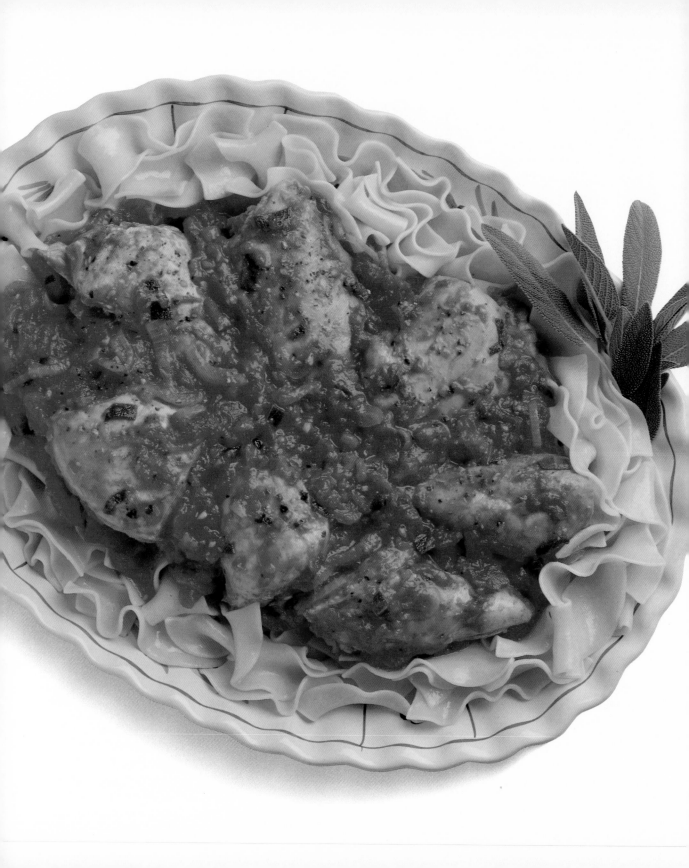

In this updated version of the popular hunter's style chicken—Italy's chicken *cacciatore*—the fat content is lowered by skinning the chicken pieces. Balsamic vinegar and a generous measure of sage enhance the flavor. Serve over wide noodles, if you like.

Tomato Sauce & Sage Stewed Chicken

Serves 8

1 roasting chicken, 4 lb (2 kg), cut into serving pieces

½ cup (4 fl oz/125 ml) Chicken Stock *(recipe on page 124)*

1 large white onion, thinly sliced

2 tablespoons Roast Garlic Sauce *(recipe on page 126)* or 2 garlic cloves, peeled and minced and mixed with 1 tablespoon white wine vinegar

2 cans (28 oz/875 g total weight) crushed tomatoes

2 cups (16 fl oz/500 ml) Quick Tomato Sauce *(recipe on page 126)*

2 tablespoons balsamic vinegar

2 tablespoons fresh sage leaves or 1 tablespoon dried sage

½–1 cup (4–8 fl oz/125–250 ml) water or Chicken Stock *(recipe on page 124)*

salt and freshly ground pepper

1. Remove the skin from the chicken pieces. Cut each chicken breast half crosswise into 3 pieces. Set aside.

2. In a heavy pot over medium-low heat, warm the Chicken Stock. Add the onion and Garlic Sauce and simmer until softened, about 5 minutes. Add the chicken pieces and continue to simmer until the chicken is golden on all sides, 5–10 minutes.

3. Stir in the crushed tomatoes, Quick Tomato Sauce, balsamic vinegar and sage. Add water or additional Chicken Stock as needed to make the dish soupier.

4. Cover partially and simmer over medium-low heat, stirring occasionally, for 30 minutes. Cut into a piece of the chicken to see if it is cooked through. Uncover and cook another 5–10 minutes if the sauce needs to thicken or the chicken needs more cooking time. Add the salt and pepper to taste and stir to mix well.

5. To serve, transfer to a warmed platter.

Nutritional Analysis Per Serving:

**CALORIES 211
(KILOJOULES 887)
PROTEIN 26 G
CARBOHYDRATES 15 G
TOTAL FAT 5 G
SATURATED FAT 1 G
CHOLESTEROL 76 MG
SODIUM 435 MG
DIETARY FIBER 3 G**

The aromatic basmati rice in this adaptation of a classic Indian *biryani* cooks faster than regular long-grain rice, but needs an initial soaking for optimum texture. Just a little clarified butter provides a touch of richness.

CURRIED CHICKEN ON SAFFRON RICE

Serves 6

2 cups (14 oz/440 g) basmati rice
2 teaspoons clarified butter or
  vegetable oil
½ teaspoon ground turmeric
1 cinnamon stick, about 3 inches
  (7.5 cm) long
3 cups (24 fl oz/750 ml) Chicken
  Stock *(recipe on page 124)*
½ teaspoon sea salt
⅛ teaspoon saffron threads, crushed
  into powder
1 large yellow onion, sliced

2 lb (1 kg) chicken thighs, skinned and
  trimmed of visible fat
2 teaspoons curry powder
2 tablespoons Roast Garlic Sauce *(recipe on
  page 126)* or 2 garlic cloves, peeled and
  minced and mixed with 1 tablespoon
  white wine vinegar
1 cup (8 oz/250 g) lowfat plain yogurt
½ green bell pepper (capsicum), seeded,
  deribbed and cut into ½-inch (12-mm)
  dice (¾ cup/4 oz/120 g)
¼ cup (¼ oz/8 g) fresh mint or cilantro
  (fresh coriander) leaves

*Nutritional Analysis
Per Serving:*

**CALORIES 398
(KILOJOULES 1,672)
PROTEIN 27 G
CARBOHYDRATES 59 G
TOTAL FAT 8 G
SATURATED FAT 2 G
CHOLESTEROL 78 MG
SODIUM 414 MG
DIETARY FIBER 2 G**

1. Place the rice in a large bowl and fill the bowl with water. Let the rice settle to the bottom of the milky water, then tilt the bowl and pour off the water. Repeat this process a few times until the water runs clear. Add 4 cups (32 fl oz/1 l) cold water to the rice in the bowl and let stand for 30 minutes. Drain.
2. Preheat an oven to 350°F (180°C).
3. In a large, heavy ovenproof pot over medium heat, warm 1 teaspoon of the butter or oil. Add the turmeric, cinnamon stick and rice and sauté for 1 minute. Add the Chicken Stock and salt and bring to a boil. Reduce the heat to low, add the saffron, cover and simmer for 10 minutes. Turn off the heat and let stand, covered, for 5 minutes.
4. While the rice is cooking, in a frying pan over medium-low heat, warm the remaining 1 teaspoon butter or oil. Add the

onion and sauté until fragrant and translucent, about 5 minutes. Add the chicken pieces and sauté, turning when the chicken colors slightly on the bottom, until lightly browned, about 10 minutes. Stir in the curry powder and Garlic Sauce and sauté for 1 minute.

5. Spoon the chicken mixture over the rice in the pot. Cover and bake until the chicken juices run clear when the chicken is pierced with a knife, about 20 minutes. Remove and discard the cinnamon sticks.

6. In a small bowl, stir together the yogurt, bell pepper and mint or cilantro.

7. To serve, place the chicken and rice on individual plates with the yogurt mixture on the side.

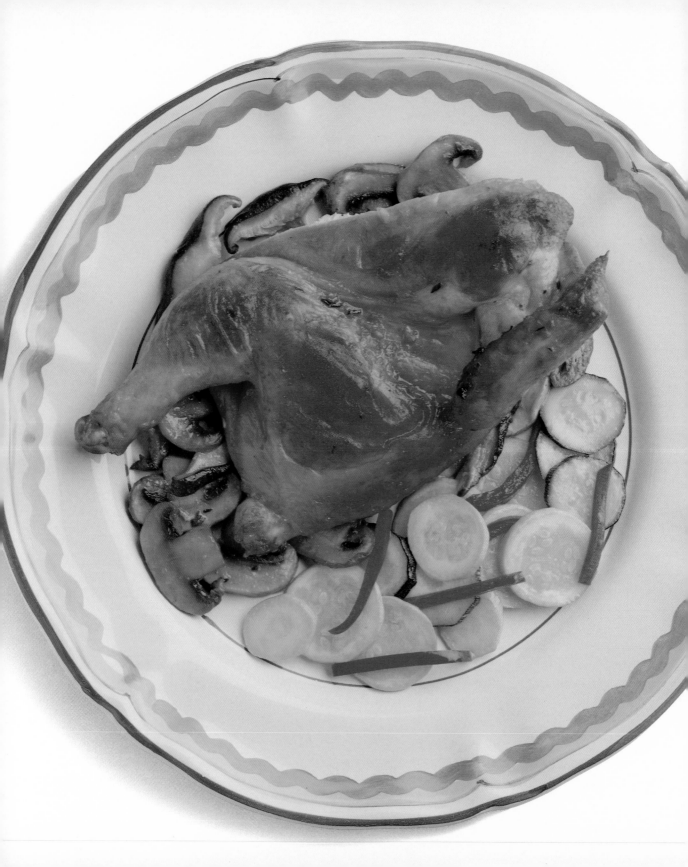

The combination of flavorful mushrooms and garlic makes this dish especially memorable. In place of the Cornish hens, you can substitute poussins, which are chickens less than 6 weeks old. If you wish to cut additional fat, remove the skin before eating.

Garlic Cornish Hens

Serves 6

3 Cornish hens
¼ cup (2 fl oz/60 ml) Roast Garlic Sauce *(recipe on page 126)* or 4 garlic cloves, peeled and minced and mixed with 2 tablespoons white wine vinegar

¼ cup (2 fl oz/60 ml) dry white wine
½ lb (250 g) fresh white cremini or shiitake mushrooms, stems removed and caps sliced

1. Preheat an oven to 425°F (220°C).

2. To split each hen, place each hen, breast-side down, on a work surface with the neck facing you. Using heavy kitchen scissors and beginning at the neck, cut down the center of the hen to the tail, then continue cutting through the backbone. Using the back of your hand, firmly press down on the breast-bone to flatten. Cut through to separate into halves. Place in a large roasting pan.

3. In a small bowl, stir together the Garlic Sauce and wine. Spoon over the hens. Tuck the mushrooms under the hens. Cover the hens with aluminum foil and roast for 10 minutes.

4. Reduce the oven temperature to 350°F (180°C). Uncover and spoon the pan juices over the hens. Continue to roast, occasionally spooning the pan juices over the hens to keep them moist, until the leg joint moves freely and the skin is crispy and golden, about 45 minutes.

5. To serve, transfer each hen half to an individual plate. Spoon an equal amount of the mushrooms and pan juices around each.

Nutritional Analysis Per Serving:

**Calories 444
(Kilojoules 1,867)
Protein 37 g
Carbohydrates 4 g
Total Fat 30 g
Saturated Fat 9 g
Cholesterol 145 mg
Sodium 138 mg
Dietary Fiber 0 g**

This quick, easy main dish offers all the flavor of a classic leg of lamb with none of the time or fuss of longer roasting. Fresh mint plays the role of the mint sauce or mint jelly that traditionally accompanies roast lamb.

ROAST LAMB CHOPS

Serves 6

6 loin lamb chops, 4 oz (125 g) each, trimmed of visible fat
2 tablespoons Roast Garlic Sauce *(recipe on page 126)* or 2 garlic cloves, peeled and minced and mixed with 1 tablespoon white wine vinegar
¼ cup (2 fl oz/60 ml) sherry vinegar
hot-pepper sauce
3 tablespoons chopped fresh mint leaves, plus the mint stems tied together with kitchen string

1. Preheat a broiler (griller).
2. Using the tip of a paring knife, cut small gashes in the meat. Brush both sides of each chop with the Garlic Sauce and place in a shallow, nonreactive dish. Marinate for 10 minutes to allow the sauce to seep into the gashes.
3. Place the chops side by side in a broiling pan. Broil (grill), turning once, until crispy brown and still pink on the inside, about 3 minutes on each side. Transfer to a warmed platter and cover to keep warm. As the juices accumulate on the platter, skim off the fat and reserve the juices.
4. Place the broiling pan on the top of the stove over low heat. When warm, stir in the sherry vinegar and hot-pepper sauce to taste. Set the mint leaves aside to use for garnish and add the stems to the pan. Scrape up any browned bits from the pan bottom and cook, stirring occasionally, until reduced and thickened, 5–8 minutes. Pour any accumulated juices from the platter into the pan.
5. To serve, remove and discard the mint stems. Place the chops on individual plates. Spoon an equal amount of the vinegar mixture over each serving and garnish with the mint leaves.

Nutritional Analysis Per Serving:

CALORIES 105
(KILOJOULES 441)
PROTEIN 13 G
CARBOHYDRATES 2 G
TOTAL FAT 5 G
SATURATED FAT 2 G
CHOLESTEROL 41 MG
SODIUM 38 MG
DIETARY FIBER 0 G

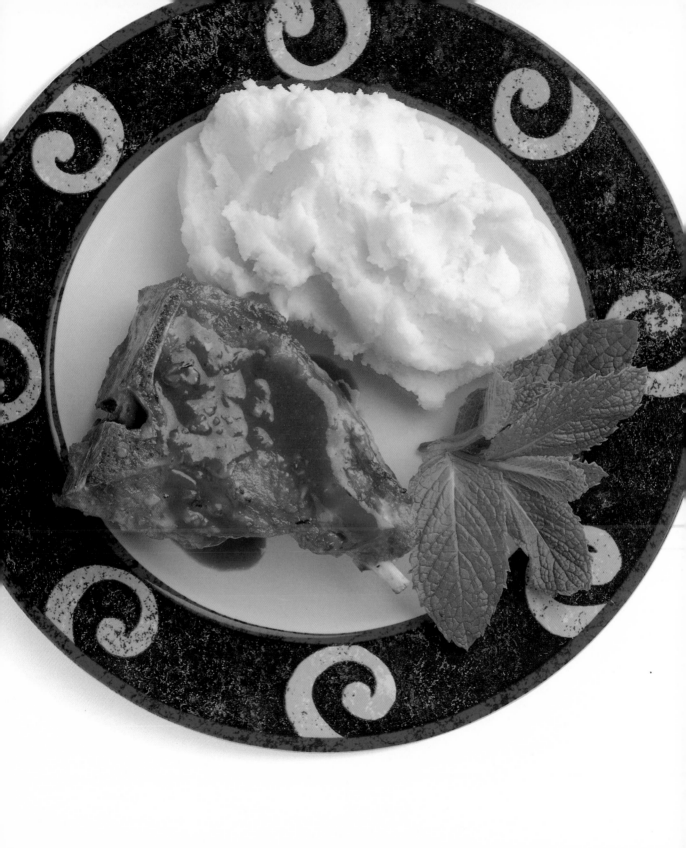

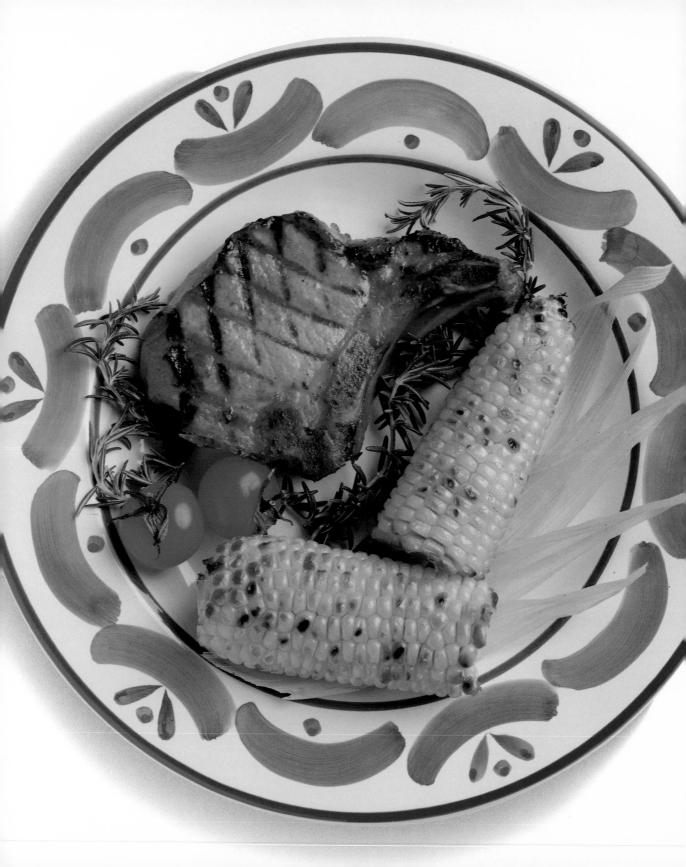

The tart edge of the cranberry juice nicely complements the sweetness of the pork chops. Be sure to trim the chops of visible fat. If you like, grill them on the barbecue, cooking them about the same amount of time as you would on top of the stove.

Pork Chops in Cranberry Mustard

Serves 4

4 pork loin chops with bone, 6 oz
  (185 g) each, trimmed of visible fat
4 teaspoons Dijon-style mustard
¼ cup (2 fl oz/60 ml) cranberry juice

1. Place the pork chops in a single layer in a shallow, nonreactive dish. In a small bowl, stir together the mustard and cranberry juice. Brush the mustard mixture evenly over the chops. Cover and refrigerate for 1 hour, turning occasionally.
2. Coat a large frying pan with nonstick cooking spray and place over medium-high heat. When the pan is hot, add the chops. Cover partially and cook 10 minutes. Uncover, turn over the chops and cook, uncovered, on the second side until the meat is cooked through but still juicy, 5–10 minutes longer.
3. To serve, transfer to individual plates.

*Nutritional Analysis
Per Serving:*

**CALORIES 185
(KILOJOULES 777)
PROTEIN 25 G
CARBOHYDRATES 3 G
TOTAL FAT 7 G
SATURATED FAT 2 G
CHOLESTEROL 68 MG
SODIUM 201 MG
DIETARY FIBER 0 G**

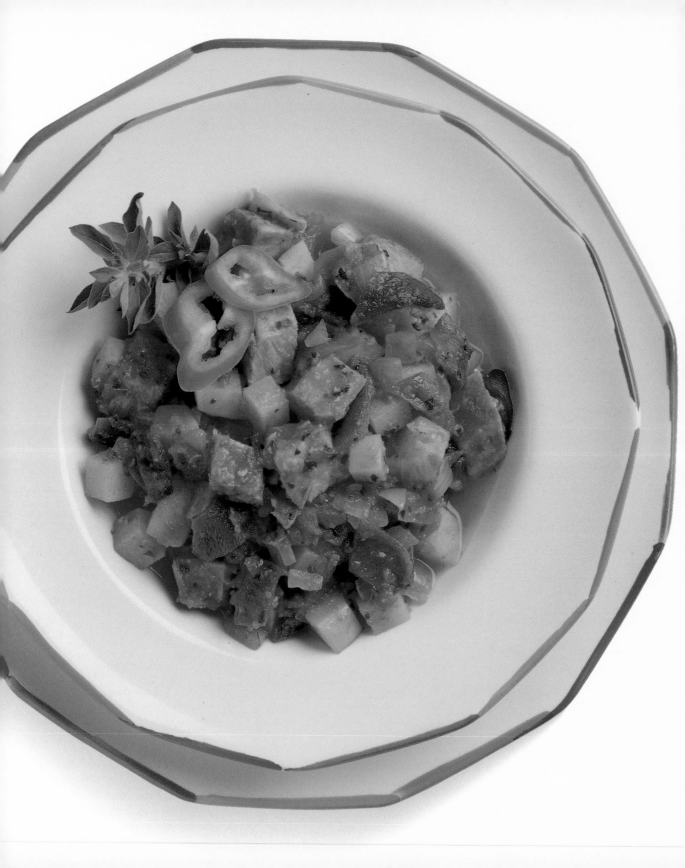

Serve this wonderful New Mexican stew on its own or tucked into warmed corn tortillas—which will add more carbohydrates to your meal. Garnish, if you like, with fresh basil. The chilies are an excellent source of vitamin C.

GREEN CHILI PORK STEW

Serves 6

1½ lb (750 g) boneless pork loin, trimmed of visible fat

⅛ teaspoon salt

⅛ teaspoon freshy ground pepper

1 cup (8 fl oz/250 ml) Vegetable Stock *(recipe on page 124)*

2 tablespoons olive oil

2 large white onions, coarsely chopped

2 teaspoons ground cumin

1 teaspoon dried oregano, crumbled, or 2 teaspoons chopped fresh oregano leaves

8 fresh poblano, Anaheim, New Mexico or other long green chili peppers, 1 lb (500 g) total weight, roasted, peeled, seeded and chopped

6 cups (48 fl oz/1.5 l) Chicken Stock or Vegetable Stock *(recipes on page 124)*

2 lb (1 kg) boiling potatoes, cut into small dice

2 cups (16 fl oz/500 ml) Quick Tomato Sauce *(recipe on page 126)*

2 teaspoons Citrus Marinade made with lime juice and tequila *(recipe on page 127)*

1. Preheat an oven to 350°F (180°C).
2. Place the pork in a shallow roasting pan. Sprinkle with the salt and pepper. Cover with the Vegetable Stock. Roast, basting occasionally with the pan drippings, until the top of the meat is brown and crispy, about 30 minutes. Cool and cut into ¾-inch (2-cm) dice.
3. In a heavy pot over medium-low heat, warm the olive oil. Add the onions, cumin and oregano and cook, stirring occasionally, until the onions are fragrant and translucent, 10–15 minutes.
4. Stir in the chili peppers, Chicken or Vegetable Stock, potatoes, Quick Tomato Sauce and pork and simmer, uncovered, until the potatoes are tender and the stew has thickened, 20–30 minutes.
5. Stir in the Citrus Marinade and simmer for 2–3 minutes to boil off the alcohol, leaving only the flavor.
6. To serve, transfer to soup plates or shallow bowls.

Nutritional Analysis Per Serving:

CALORIES 523 (KILOJOULES 2,197)
PROTEIN 41 G
CARBOHYDRATES 49 G
TOTAL FAT 19 G
SATURATED FAT 5 G
CHOLESTEROL 92 MG
SODIUM 461 MG
DIETARY FIBER 2 G

For the best flavor, use spicy apples such as Empire, McIntosh or late-season Winesaps. Apple cider, available fresh in the fall, can be frozen for later use. Because the sauce separates as it cools, serve this dish as soon as you take it from the oven.

Pork Tenderloin Medallions

Serves 6

6 spicy apples, quartered, cored and thinly sliced

2 celery stalks, diced

1 leek, white part only, carefully washed and thinly sliced

¾ cup (6 fl oz/180 ml) fresh unfiltered apple cider

1 tablespoon unsalted butter

3 boneless pork loin chops, 8 oz (250 g) each, trimmed of visible fat and cut in half

1 cup (8 fl oz/250 ml) Chicken Stock *(recipe on page 124)*

freshly grated nutmeg

2 tablespoons nonfat plain yogurt

Nutritional Analysis Per Serving:

Calories 277

(Kilojoules 1,162)

Protein 23 g

Carbohydrates 29 g

Total Fat 8 g

Saturated Fat 3 g

Cholesterol 68 mg

Sodium 140 mg

Dietary Fiber 4 g

1. Preheat an oven to 400°F (200°C). Coat a 2-qt (2-l) baking dish with nonstick cooking spray.

2. Spread the apples, celery and leek in the prepared dish. Drizzle with ¼ cup (2 fl oz/60 ml) of the apple cider. Bake uncovered for 15 minutes.

3. Meanwhile, in a nonstick frying pan over medium heat, melt the butter. Add the pork chops and cook, turning once, until nicely browned, 8 minutes on each side. Place the chops atop the apples and vegetables in the baking dish and set aside.

4. Add the remaining ½ cup (4 fl oz/120 ml) cider and Chicken Stock to the frying pan and cook, uncovered, over medium-high heat, scraping up any browned bits on the pan bottom, until the liquid is reduced by half, 10–15 minutes.

5. Pour the sauce evenly over the chops. Shake the dish gently so the sauce penetrates the bed of apples and vegetables. Sprinkle nutmeg to taste over the top. Return the dish to the oven and bake until warmed through, about 15 minutes longer.

6. Transfer each chop to an individual plate. Swirl the yogurt into the mixture in the baking dish.

7. To serve, pour an equal amount of the mixture over each chop.

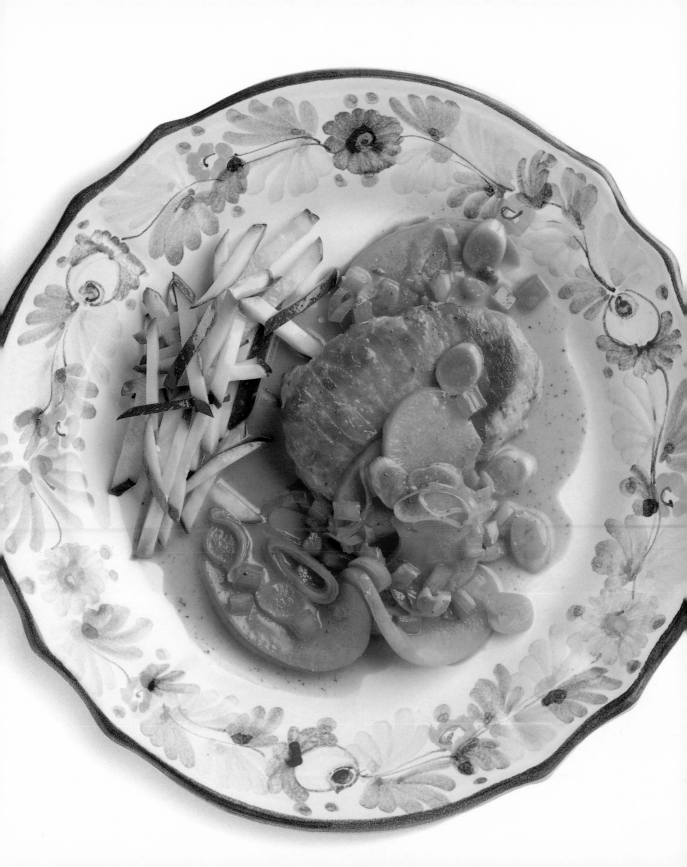

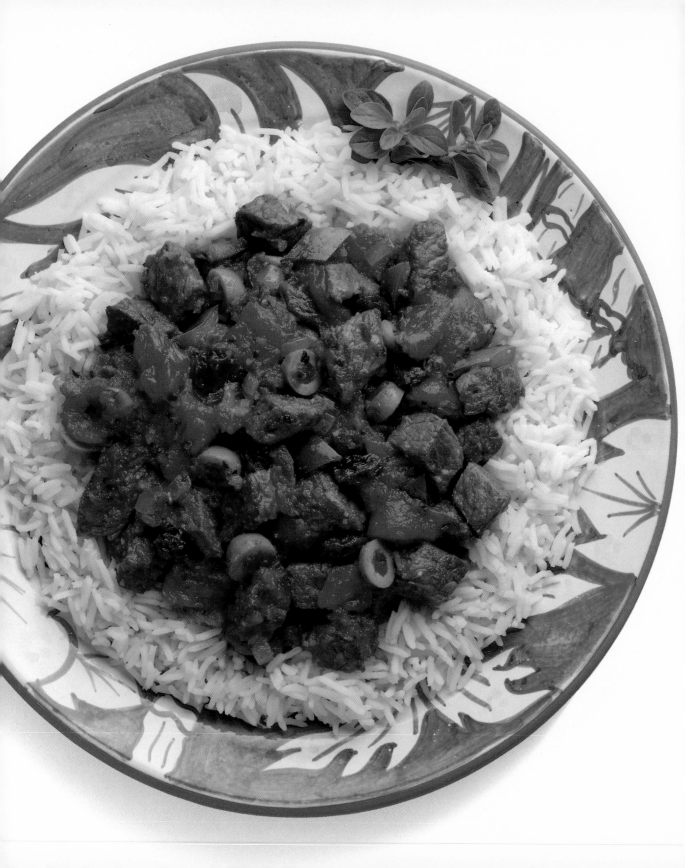

Known as *picadillo* in its native Cuba, this spicy hash blends beef and tomatoes with the sweet punch of cinnamon and raisins. Use cubes of top round steak, a fairly lowfat cut, or, to lower the fat further still, substitute cubed turkey breast.

CUBAN-STYLE HASH

Serves 6

3 cups (24 fl oz/750 ml) water
1½ cups (10½ oz/330 g) white rice
1 tablespoon vegetable oil
1 lb (500 g) lean beef, cut into
 1-inch (2.5-cm) cubes
1 teaspoon dried ground chili
1 white onion, finely chopped
1 green bell pepper (capsicum),
 seeded, deribbed and diced
2 teaspoons dried oregano

2 tablespoons Roast Garlic Sauce *(recipe on page 126)* or 2 garlic cloves, peeled and minced and mixed with 1 tablespoon white wine vinegar
1 can (14½ oz/455 g) stewed tomatoes, with their juices
2 cups (16 fl oz/500 ml) Quick Tomato Sauce *(recipe on page 126)*
½ cup (2½ oz/75 g) green olives, stuffed with pimiento, halved crosswise
¼ cup (1½ oz/45 g) raisins

1. In a medium saucepan, bring the water to a boil. Stir in the rice, lower the heat and simmer, covered, for 18 minutes. Turn off the heat and let sit until the hash is cooked.

2. In a heavy saucepan over medium heat, warm the vegetable oil and brown the meat, about 5 minutes. Drain off and discard all but 1 tablespoon of the fat. Sprinkle the meat with the chili powder, transfer to a plate and reserve.

3. In the same pan, combine the onion, bell pepper, oregano and Garlic Sauce with the small amount of remaining fat. Cook over medium heat, stirring occasionally, until the onions are fragrant and translucent, about 5 minutes.

4. Stir in the reserved meat, stewed tomatoes, Quick Tomato Sauce and olives. Cook, uncovered, stirring occasionally, for 10 minutes. Stir in the raisins and cook to blend the flavors, 5 minutes longer.

5. To serve, spoon the hash over the rice.

Nutritional Analysis Per Serving:

**CALORIES 393
(KILOJOULES 1,650)
PROTEIN 22 G
CARBOHYDRATES 56 G
TOTAL FAT 9 G
SATURATED FAT 2 G
CHOLESTEROL 45 MG
SODIUM 510 MG
DIETARY FIBER 4 G**

One of the leaner beef cuts, flank has a satisfying taste and texture that make a little go a long way. Here, it is complemented by a bourbon-laced barbecue sauce. For a smoky flavor, add fragrant wood chips such as hickory, apple or pecan to the fire.

Glazed Flank Steak

Serves 6

½ cup (4 fl oz/125 ml) bourbon whiskey

¾ cup (6 fl oz/180 ml) Quick Tomato Sauce *(recipe on page 126)*

¼ cup (2 fl oz/60 ml) dark corn syrup

2 tablespoons peanut oil

1 tablespoon Roast Garlic Sauce *(recipe on page 126)* or 1 garlic clove, peeled and minced and mixed with 2 teaspoons white wine vinegar

1 star anise

1 flank steak, 1½ lb (750 g) and ½ inch (12 mm) thick, trimmed of visible fat

Nutritional Analysis Per Serving:

CALORIES 317
(KILOJOULES 1,330)
PROTEIN 23 G
CARBOHYDRATES 12 G
TOTAL FAT 14 G
SATURATED FAT 5 G
CHOLESTEROL 57 MG
SODIUM 95 MG
DIETARY FIBER 0 G

1. In a shallow glass nonreactive pan or dish large enough to hold the steak flat, stir together the bourbon, Quick Tomato Sauce, corn syrup, peanut oil, Garlic Sauce and star anise.

2. If the steak is thicker than ½ inch (12 mm), flatten it by pounding with the edge of a plate or meat mallet. Using a sharp knife, score it in a diamond pattern on each side, cutting about ⅛ inch (3 mm) deep so the meat won't curl during cooking. Slip the steak into the marinade. Turn to coat evenly. Cover and refrigerate overnight.

3. Prepare a fire in a charcoal grill or preheat a broiler (griller).

4. Drain off the marinade into a small saucepan. Bring to a boil and cook for 5 minutes. Cover and keep warm over low heat.

5. Place the steak on the grill or broiler rack and cook, turning once, until done to your liking, about 3 minutes on each side for medium rare.

6. To serve, carve the meat on the diagonal and arrange on individual plates. Pour an equal amount of the marinade over each portion.

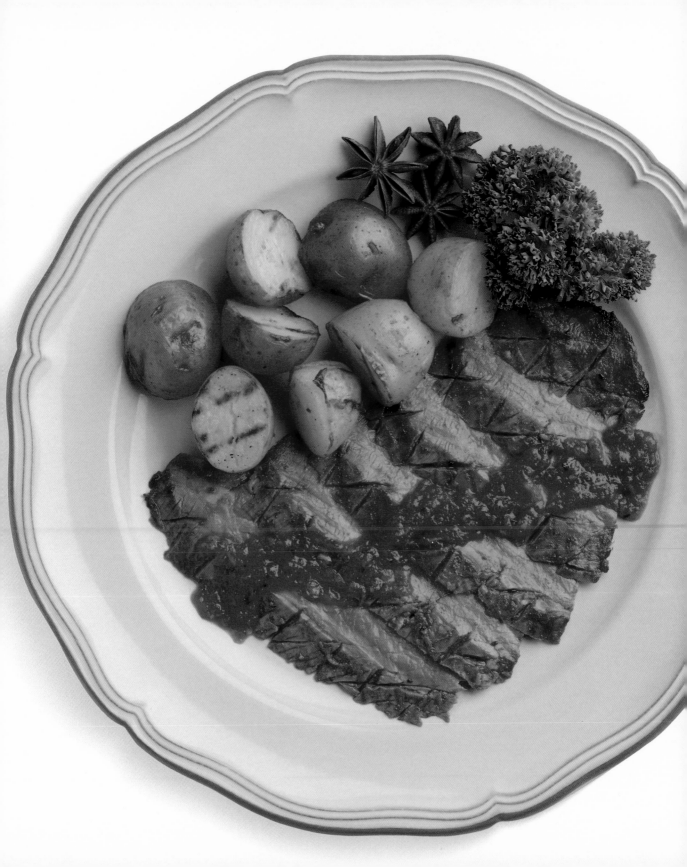

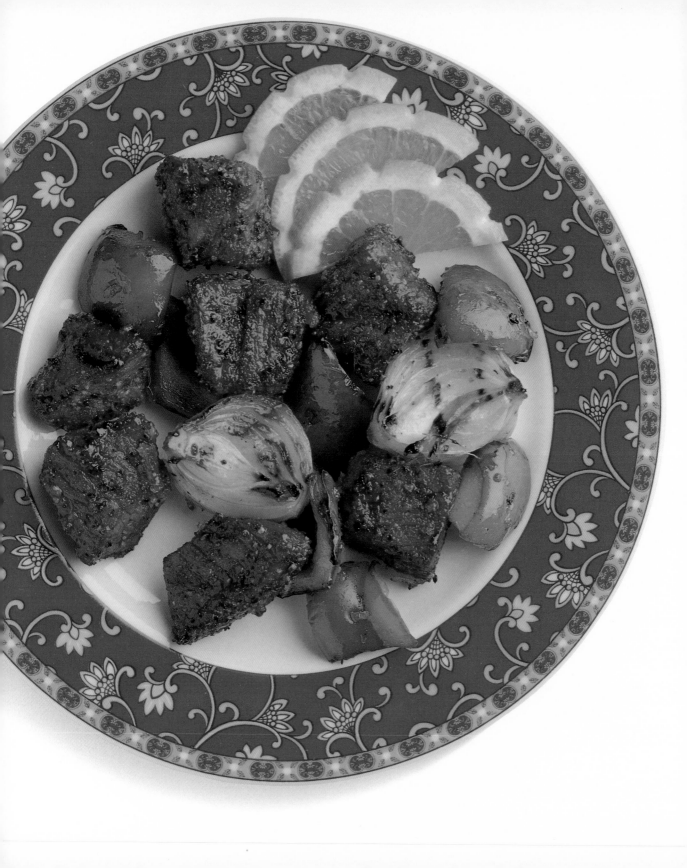

Chunks of vegetables literally stretch out the steak in these main dish skewers. If Vidalia onions aren't available, seek out another sweet variety such as Maui or Walla Walla. Try the delicious orange glaze on steaks or pork loins as well as kabobs.

Orange-Glazed Beef Kabobs

Serves 6

1 tablespoon coarsely ground
  pepper
1½ lb (750 g) New York strip
  steak, trimmed of visible fat and
  cut into 1-inch (2.5-cm) cubes
3 large Vidalia onions, quartered

2 green bell peppers (capsicums),
  seeded, deribbed and cut into
  1-inch (2.5-cm) pieces
⅓ cup (3½ oz/105 g) orange marmalade
1 tablespoon cider vinegar
½ teaspoon grated, peeled fresh ginger

1. Prepare a fire in a charcoal grill or preheat a broiler (griller). Away from the fire, coat the grill rack with nonstick cooking spray.

2. Put the ground pepper in a shallow bowl and press the beef chunks into the pepper to cover the meat evenly. Alternately thread the beef, onions and pepper pieces onto 6 skewers. In a small bowl, stir together the marmalade, cider vinegar and ginger. Brush the meat cubes on one side with the marmalade mixture.

3. Place the skewers on the grill or broiler rack, brushed side up, and cook, turning once or twice and brushing with more marmalade mixture, about 8 minutes' total cooking time for medium.

4. To serve, pull the beef, onion and peppers from the skewers and place on individual plates.

Nutritional Analysis Per Serving:

**Calories 299
(Kilojoules 1,257)
Protein 28 g
Carbohydrates 30 g
Total Fat 8 g
Saturated Fat 3 g
Cholesterol 65 mg
Sodium 87 mg
Dietary Fiber 3 g**

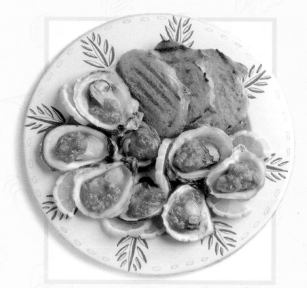

Fish & Shellfish

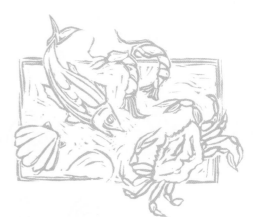

Seafood presents the home cook with a more varied range of choices than virtually any other category of main dish in-gredients. Delicate trout and snapper; sweet, succulent shrimp and crab; meaty tuna, swordfish and salmon; succulent mussels, clams and oysters: These and dozens of other kinds of seafood presented on the following pages await your culinary enjoyment. The pleasure such a broad selection offers becomes all the greater in light of seafood's proven health benefits. Packed with protein, seafood is generally lower in fat than meat or poultry and certain fattier varieties, such as tuna and salmon, contain rich amounts of the omega-3 oils that have been found to help prevent heart disease. The recipes that follow reflect a long-standing, worldwide tradition of sea-food cuisine, with recipes inspired by the local dishes of the Caribbean islands, Italy, India, France, Japan, Mexico, Vietnam

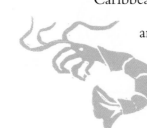

and other points on the compass. Most can be readily adapted to the seasonally fresh fish substitutes available in your area (see page 11).

This main course gains a haunting flavor from lemongrass and fish sauce, both available in Asian markets and well-stocked food stores. Grated orange zest may be used in place of lemongrass. Substitute any firm, meaty fish such as tuna or bluefish.

SWORDFISH SIMMERED IN FISH SAUCE

Serves 6

2 tablespoons peanut oil

2 green (spring) onions, thinly sliced

1 fresh jalapeño or other chili pepper, seeded and minced

2 tablespoons Roast Garlic Sauce *(recipe on page 126)* or 2 garlic cloves, peeled and minced and mixed with 1 tablespoon white wine vinegar

¼ cup (2 fl oz/60 ml) fish sauce

1 piece lemongrass stalk, 3 inches (7.5 cm) long, outer husk removed and slit open lengthwise, or 2 teaspoons ground lemongrass

3 cups (24 fl oz/750 ml) water

1 large lime, thinly sliced

1 teaspoon sugar

1½ lb (750 g) swordfish steaks, cut into 1-inch (2.5-cm) pieces

1. In a large frying pan or heavy pot over medium heat, warm the oil. Add the green onions and jalapeño or chili pepper and sauté, stirring, for 1 minute. Stir in the Garlic Sauce and sauté for 30 seconds longer.

2. Add the fish sauce, lemongrass, water, lime and sugar. When the liquid is simmering, add the swordfish. Simmer, uncovered, until the fish is opaque when pierced with a knife, about 8 minutes. Remove and discard the lemongrass stalk.

3. To serve, place the fish in shallow bowls. Top with the aromatic liquid.

Nutritional Analysis Per Serving:

CALORIES 207

(KILOJOULES 870)

PROTEIN 22 G

CARBOHYDRATES 6 G

TOTAL FAT 10 G

SATURATED FAT 2 G

CHOLESTEROL 40 MG

SODIUM 93 MG

DIETARY FIBER 0 G

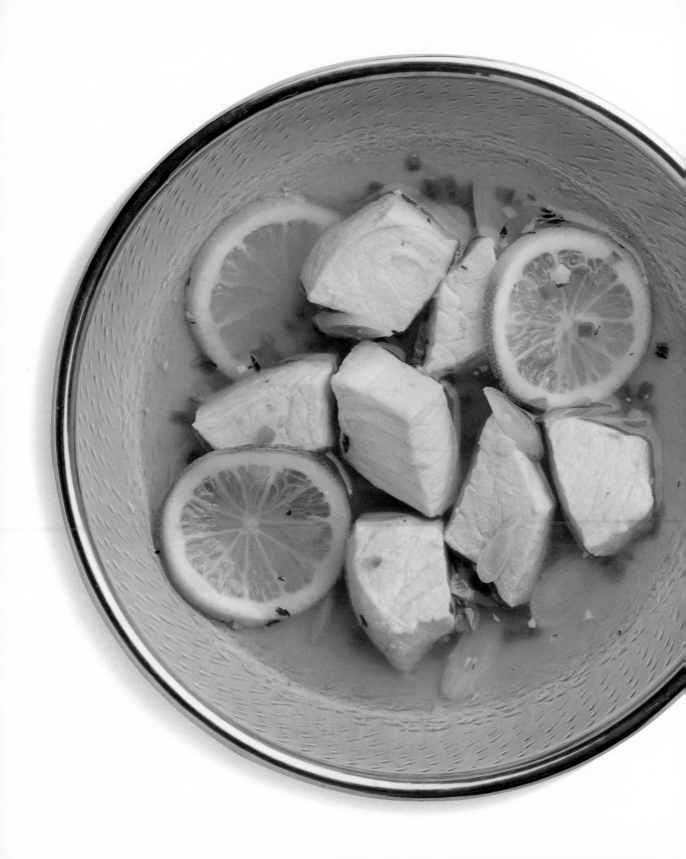

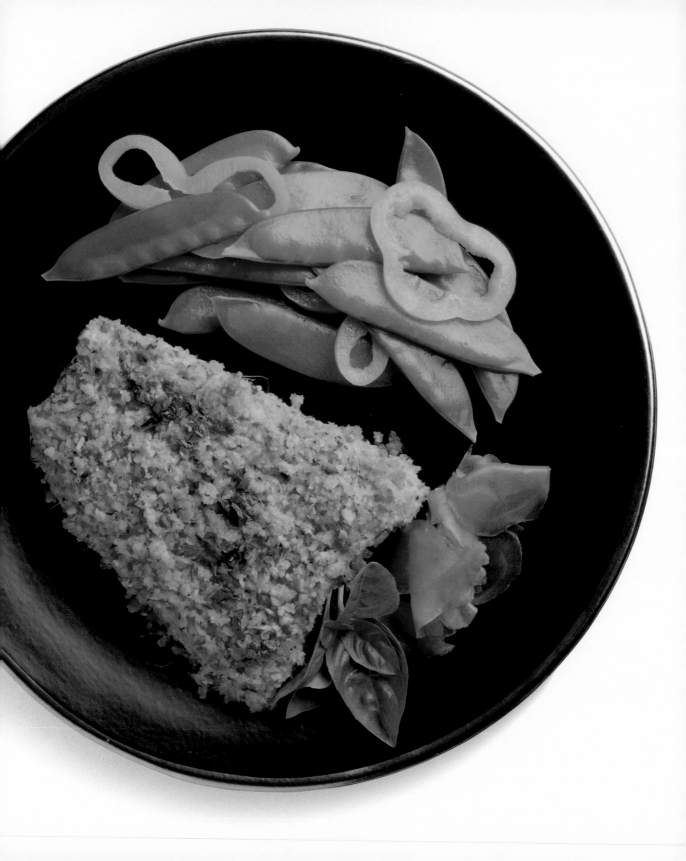

Lighter than a conventional vinaigrette, the mixture of rice vinegar and sesame oil provides a pleasant spark of flavor when added just before serving. If fresh salmon is unavailable, try this recipe with halibut or sea bass.

CRUMB-CRUSTED SALMON

Serves 6

2 tablespoons grated, peeled fresh ginger

2 tablespoons Nut Crumbs made with almonds *(recipe on page 125)*

½ cup (2 oz/60 g) Seasoned Bread Crumbs *(recipe on page 125)*

3 salmon fillets or steaks, 8 oz (250 g) each, halved

2 tablespoons rice wine vinegar

1 tablespoon fresh orange juice or dry sherry

1 teaspoon miso or 1 tablespoon low-sodium soy sauce

2 teaspoons Flavored Sesame Oil *(recipe on page 127)*

2 tablespoons fresh basil leaves, finely chopped

6 tablespoons (3 oz/90 g) well-drained pickled ginger

1. Preheat an oven to 400°F (200°C).

2. In a small bowl, stir together the grated ginger, Nut Crumbs and Seasoned Bread Crumbs. Press the mixture evenly into both sides of each salmon fillet. Place the fillets in a single layer in a baking dish.

3. Bake for 7 minutes. Turn the fillets over and bake until the fish is opaque when pierced with a knife, 3–5 minutes longer. Do not overcook or the fish will be dry.

4. Meanwhile, in a small bowl combine the rice wine vinegar, orange juice or sherry, miso or soy sauce, Flavored Sesame Oil and basil.

5. To serve, place a fillet and 1 tablespoon pickled ginger on each plate. Drizzle each fillet with an equal amount of the vinaigrette and serve immediately.

Nutritional Analysis Per Serving:

**CALORIES 217
(KILOJOULES 911)
PROTEIN 24 G
CARBOHYDRATES 5 G
TOTAL FAT 11 G
SATURATED FAT 2 G
CHOLESTEROL 62 MG
SODIUM 156 MG
DIETARY FIBER 0 G**

Mahi mahi is a firm, sweet-flavored fish that flakes into large pieces when broken with a fork. The fillets are easily skinned: Simply slide a sharp knife between the skin and flesh and peel the skin away. Red snapper may be substituted.

Mahi Mahi & Vegetables in Parchment

Serves 6

1½ lb (750 g) mahi mahi fillets, skin removed and cut into 1-inch (2.5-cm) cubes

⅛ teaspoon sea salt

⅛ teaspoon freshly ground pepper

2 leeks, white part only, carefully washed and thinly sliced

2 yellow bell peppers (capsicums), seeded, deribbed and cut into long, narrow strips

1 sweet potato, peeled and cut into small dice

1 lb (500 g) green Swiss chard (silverbeet), stalks cut into long, narrow strips and leaves cut into wide ribbons

1 cup (1 oz/30 g) cilantro (fresh coriander) leaves

¾ cup (6 fl oz/180 ml) sweet vermouth

2 tablespoons rice wine vinegar

2 tablespoons olive oil

2 tablespoons Quick Tomato Sauce *(recipe on page 126)*

Nutritional Analysis Per Serving:

Calories 232
(Kilojoules 974)
Protein 24 g
Carbohydrates 19 g
Total Fat 6 g
Saturated Fat 1 g
Cholesterol 83 mg
Sodium 307 mg
Dietary Fiber 2 g

1. Preheat an oven to 400°F (200°C). Coat a large roasting pan with nonstick cooking spray.

2. Working from a narrow end, fold six 24-by-16-inch (60-by-40-cm) pieces of parchment paper or aluminum foil in half. Using scissors and starting at the fold, cut out half of a heart as large as possible. Open the papers to reveal full hearts and lay them out flat on a work surface.

3. Arrange an equal portion of the fish on half of each heart. Sprinkle with the salt and pepper. Top each with an equal amount of the leeks, bell peppers, sweet potato, Swiss chard and cilantro leaves. Drizzle the vermouth and rice wine vinegar over the top. Fold over the other half of the heart. Roll up the edges of each heart so they are airtight and secure. Place in the roasting pan. Bake for 25 minutes.

4. In a small bowl, mix the olive oil and Quick Tomato Sauce.

5. To serve, place the packets on individual plates. Drizzle 2 teaspoons of the oil mixture atop the fish and vegetables.

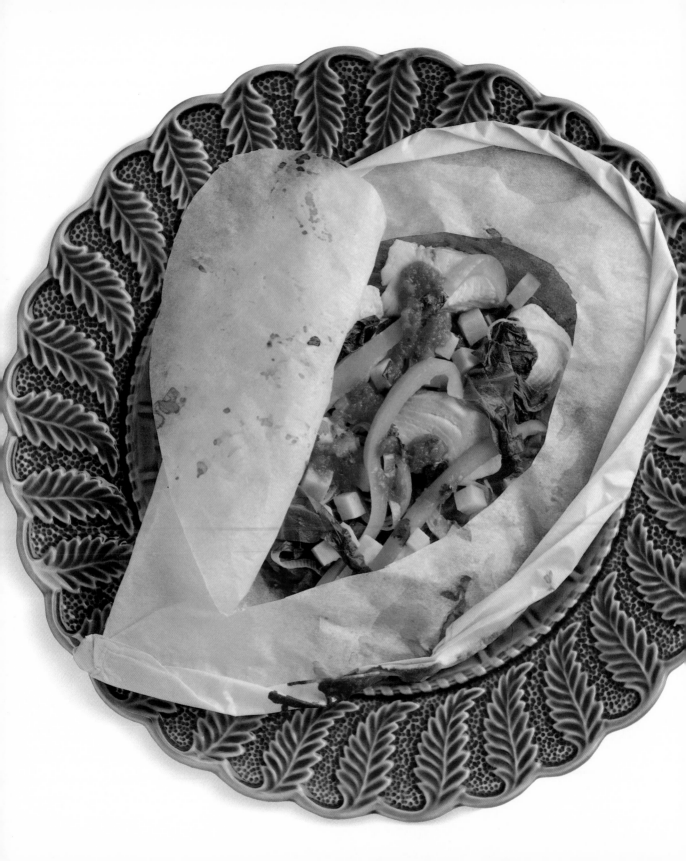

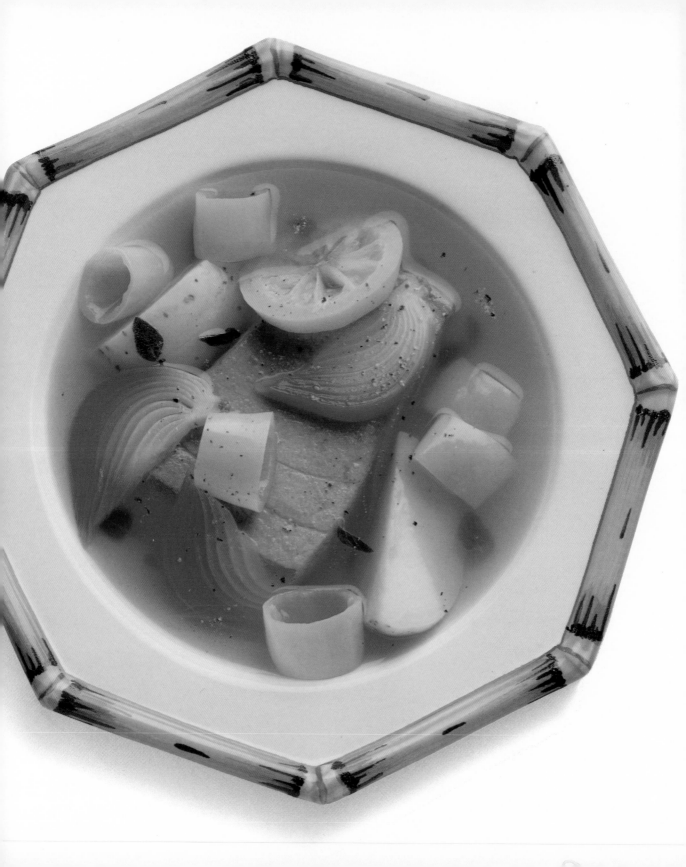

Anchovy paste contributes robust flavor to this dish, and, because it is salty, only a fairly small amount is necessary. In place of the tuna, you can substitute any firm, lean fish, such as swordfish, sea bass or bluefish.

Garlic- & Anchovy-Studded Tuna

Serves 6

1 tablespoon anchovy paste
¼ cup (2 fl oz/60 ml) Roast Garlic Sauce *(recipe on page 126)* or 4 garlic cloves, peeled and minced and mixed with 2 tablespoons white wine vinegar
6 tuna steaks, 4 oz (125 g) each
2 red (Spanish) onions, cut into wedges
3 white boiling potatoes

6 fresh sweet banana peppers or Hungarian wax peppers, seeded and cut into rings 1 inch (2.5 cm) wide
1 cup (8 fl oz/250 ml) dry white wine
1 lemon, thickly sliced and seeded
2 cups (16 fl oz/500 ml) Vegetable Stock *(recipe on page 124)* or water
¼ teaspoon freshly ground pepper
1 teaspoon dried oregano or 2 teaspoons fresh oregano leaves
½ lb (250 g) sourdough bread, sliced

1. In a small bowl, stir together the anchovy paste and Garlic Sauce. Using the point of a sharp paring knife, cut several small slits into each steak. Press the anchovy mixture into the slits.
2. Place the onions, potatoes and fresh peppers in a large, wide, heavy pot. Pour in the wine, lemon slices and Vegetable Stock or water. Sprinkle with the pepper and oregano. Bring to a simmer, cover and cook over medium-low heat until the vegetables are very tender and the liquid is aromatic, about 20 minutes.
3. Add the tuna steaks; there should be ample liquid in the pot to cover the steaks by 1 inch (2.5 cm) or more. Cover and simmer over medium-low heat until the fish is cooked through, about 10 minutes.
4. To serve, place the tuna steaks into soup plates or shallow bowls. Spoon the vegetable mixture and liquid over the top. Use the bread for dipping.

Nutritional Analysis Per Serving:

**Calories 375
(Kilojoules 1,576)
Protein 32 g
Carbohydrates 46 g
Total Fat 8 g
Saturated Fat 2 g
Cholesterol 40 mg
Sodium 400 mg
Dietary Fiber 4 g**

The robust flavor of tuna stands up well to a rich, aromatic marinade that features miso, a fermented soybean paste available in Asian markets and well-stocked food stores. Other meaty fish, such as swordfish, sea bass and bluefish, may be substituted.

GRILLED TUNA IN MISO MARINADE

Serves 6

¼ cup (2 fl oz/60 ml) rice wine vinegar

¼ cup (2 fl oz/60 ml) sake

2 tablespoons miso or low-sodium soy sauce

2 tablespoons grated, unpeeled fresh ginger

1 red (Spanish) onion, cut into thin wedges

1 tablespoon walnut oil

6 tuna steaks, 4 oz (125 g) each

1. Prepare a fire in a charcoal grill or preheat a broiler (griller). Away from the fire, coat the grill rack with nonstick cooking spray.

2. In a large, shallow, nonreactive dish, combine the rice wine vinegar, sake, miso or soy sauce and ginger. Put the tuna steaks in the dish and turn to coat with the marinade. Let stand at room temperature for 30 minutes, or cover and refrigerate for 2 hours. Bring the tuna to room temperature before grilling.

3. Brush the onion wedges with the walnut oil and place in a hinged basket on the grill or on a baking sheet under the broiler. Cook, turning and shaking them occasionally, until softened and lightly browned, about 10 minutes.

4. Place the tuna steaks on the grill or broiler rack and cook, turning once and brushing frequently with the marinade, until the meat turns white and is firm to the touch, 3–5 minutes on each side. Do not overcook or the fish will be dry.

5. To serve, transfer the tuna steaks and onions to individual plates.

Nutritional Analysis Per Serving:

CALORIES 200

(KILOJOULES 838)

PROTEIN 25 G

CARBOHYDRATES 5 G

TOTAL FAT 8 G

SATURATED FAT 2 G

CHOLESTEROL 38 MG

SODIUM 254 MG

DIETARY FIBER 1 G

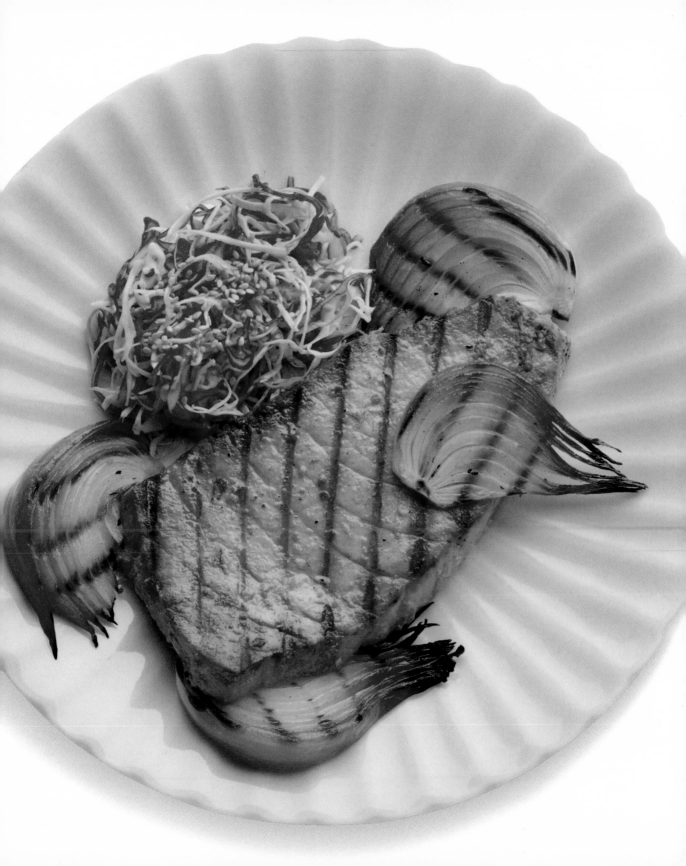

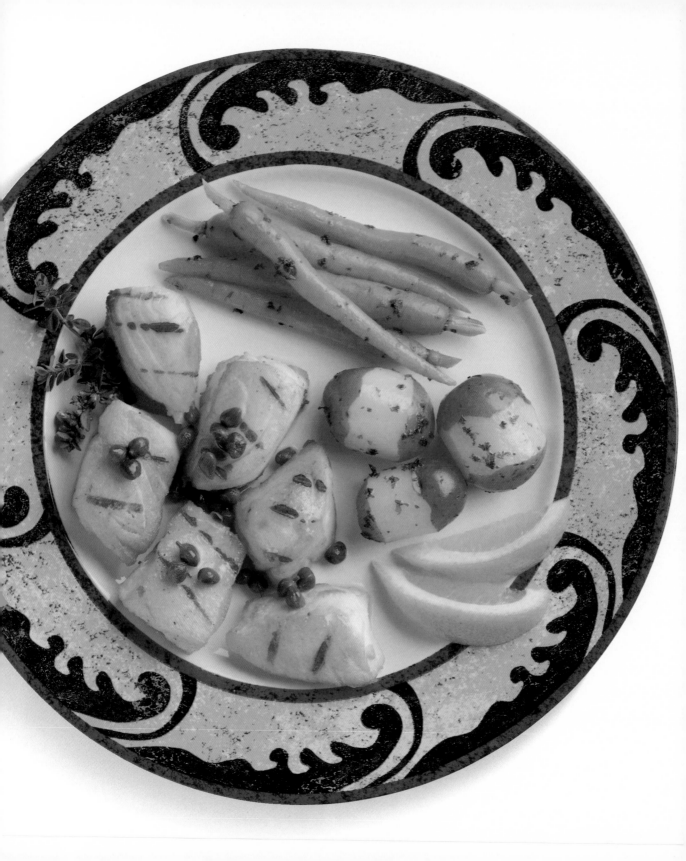

Chunks of barbecued halibut have an incredibly full flavor—the result of an aromatic combination of capers, sherry, lemon and thyme. Substitute sturgeon or salmon for the halibut, if necessary. Presoak wooden skewers in water for 30 minutes to prevent burning.

GRILLED HALIBUT BROCHETTES

Serves 6

¼ cup (2 oz/60 g) well-drained capers

¼ cup (2 fl oz/60 ml) dry sherry

1½ lbs (750 g) halibut steaks, cut into 2-inch (5-cm) cubes

2 tablespoons olive oil

¼ cup (2 fl oz/60 ml) fresh lemon juice

2 lemons, each cut into 6 wedges

6 fresh thyme or lemon thyme sprigs

1. Prepare a fire in a charcoal grill or preheat an oven to 400°F (200°C). Away from the fire, coat the grill rack with nonstick cooking spray.

2. In a small bowl, combine the capers and sherry and set aside.

3. Brush the fish pieces with the olive oil and thread them onto the skewers. Place the skewers on the grill rack or in a shallow roasting pan in the oven. Cook, turning the skewers a few times, until the fish is opaque when pierced with a knife, 6–8 minutes on the grill or 8–10 minutes in the oven.

4. While the fish is cooking, make the sauce. Drain the capers, reserving the sherry. In a saucepan over medium heat, warm the reserved sherry and the lemon juice. Stir in the capers and cook 1 minute longer.

5. To serve, slide the brochettes from the skewers onto individual plates. Top with equal amounts of the sherry mixture. Garnish each plate with 2 lemon wedges and a thyme sprig.

Nutritional Analysis Per Serving:

CALORIES 171 (KILOJOULES 719)
PROTEIN 20 G
CARBOHYDRATES 7 G
TOTAL FAT 7 G
SATURATED FAT 1 G
CHOLESTEROL 29 MG
SODIUM 199 MG
DIETARY FIBER 0 G

Sea bass fillets are meaty enough to support robust seasonings as well as the slow simmering of braising. Herb stems, used here, round out the flavor of the sauce; save the leaves for other recipes. Mahi mahi, monkfish, grouper or tuna may be substituted.

Sea Bass in Tomato-Fennel Sauce

Serves 6

2 fennel bulbs, 12 oz (375 g) total weight, with stems and fronds intact

2 tablespoons olive oil

1 yellow onion, chopped

3 sea bass fillets, 8 oz (250 g) each, halved

⅛ teaspoon sea salt

⅛ teaspoon freshly ground pepper

½ cup (4 fl oz/125 ml) Roast Garlic Sauce *(recipe on page 126)* or 8 garlic cloves, peeled and minced and mixed with ¼ cup (2 fl oz/60 ml) white wine vinegar

2 cups (16 fl oz/500 ml) Vegetable Stock *(recipe on page 124)* or water

2 cups (16 fl oz/500 ml) Quick Tomato Sauce *(recipe on page 126)*

½ cup (4 fl oz/125 ml) vermouth or dry white wine

1 can (14½ oz/455 g) stewed tomatoes

2 tablespoons well-drained capers

½ cup (2½ oz/75 g) pitted, drained and chopped green olives

1 lemon, cut into thin slices

Nutritional Analysis Per Serving:

Calories 296

(Kilojoules 1,243)

Protein 25 g

Carbohydrates 20 g

Total Fat 12 g

Saturated Fat 2 g

Cholesterol 46 mg

Sodium 695 mg

Dietary Fiber 4 g

1. Remove the fronds and stems from the fennel bulbs. Finely chop the fronds and finely dice the stems. Remove and discard the outer leaves of the bulbs. Cut the bulbs lengthwise into long, thin strips.

2. In a large heavy pot over medium heat, warm the olive oil. Add the onion and fennel strips and sauté, stirring, until all are fragrant and translucent, about 10 minutes.

3. Push the onion and fennel to one side. Add the fish fillets, salt and pepper. Sauté until the fish starts to firm up, 3–4 minutes.

4. Stir in the Garlic Sauce, Vegetable Stock or water, Quick Tomato Sauce, vermouth or wine, tomatoes, capers, olives and lemon. Bring to a boil, reduce the heat to medium-low, cover and simmer until the fish is opaque when pierced with a knife, about 10 minutes.

5. To serve, transfer the fish and sauce to individual plates. Sprinkle with the fennel fronds.

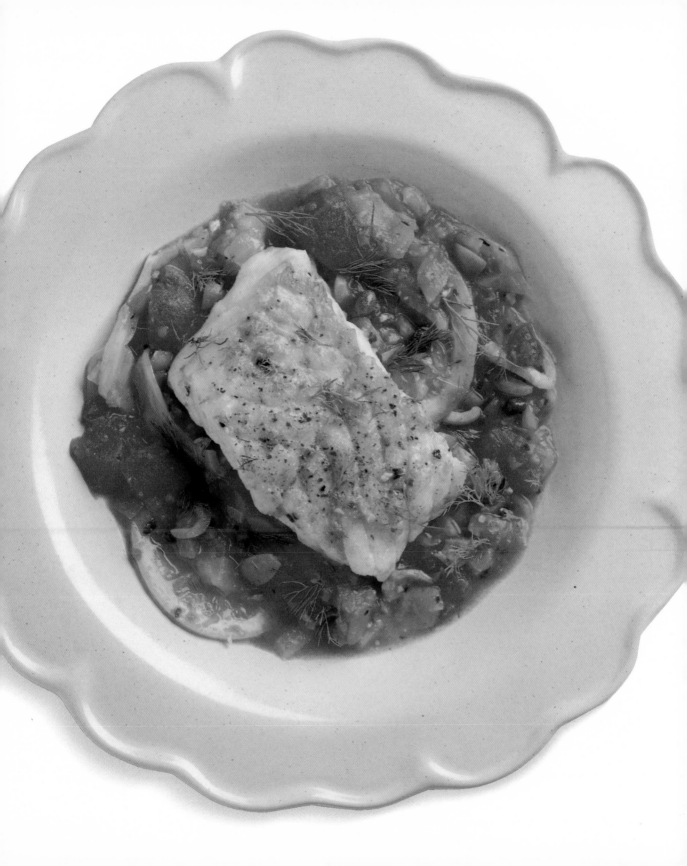

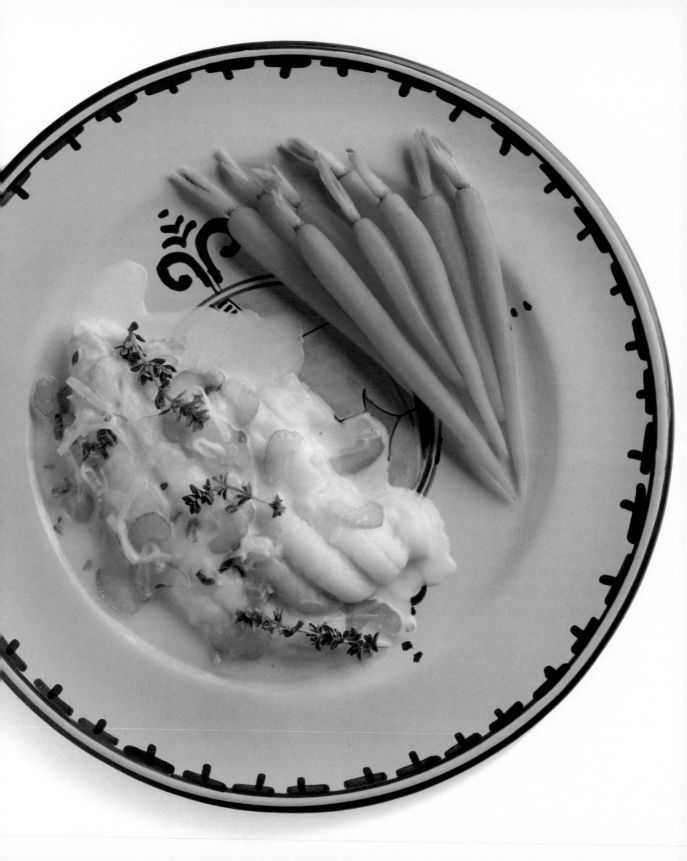

Lowfat milk tenderizes and sweetens the mild white flesh of sole, forming a lovely herb-flecked sauce as the liquid reduces during cooking. Other delicately textured fish such as flounder or tilapia (tile fish) may be substituted.

Milk-Simmered Sole

Serves 6

¼ cup (2 oz/60 g) unsalted butter
3 leeks, white part only, carefully washed and thinly sliced
8 fresh lemon thyme or thyme sprigs
2 celery stalks, including leaves, thinly sliced

2 cups (16 fl oz/500 ml) lowfat milk
6 sole fillets, 6 oz (185 g) each
⅛ teaspoon salt
⅛ teaspoon freshly ground pepper
¼ cup (2 fl oz/60 ml) dry white wine
1 tablespoon cornstarch (cornflour)

1. Preheat an oven to 350°F (180°C).
2. Place a 2-qt (2-l) flameproof baking pan on the stove top over medium-low heat and melt the butter in it. Add the leeks, half of the lemon thyme sprigs and the celery, cover partially and cook, stirring occasionally, for 10 minutes. Stir in the milk and remove from the heat.
3. Lay the sole fillets on top of the vegetables in the pan and then press on them to immerse them in the milk. Sprinkle evenly with the salt and pepper.
4. Place in the oven and bake, spooning a little of the pan juices over the fillets once or twice, until the fish is opaque throughout when pierced with a knife, about 15 minutes.
5. Remove the dish from the oven. Using a slotted spatula, transfer the fillets, leeks and celery to a warmed platter. Keep warm. Remove and discard the thyme sprigs. Place the pan on the stove top over medium heat and bring to a simmer.
6. In a small bowl, whisk together the wine and cornstarch and stir into the pan. Simmer until thickened, about 30 seconds.
7. To serve, spoon the sauce over the fish and garnish with the remaining lemon thyme sprigs.

Nutritional Analysis Per Serving:

CALORIES 309
(KILOJOULES 1,298)
PROTEIN 36 G
CARBOHYDRATES 15 G
TOTAL FAT 11 G
SATURATED FAT 6 G
CHOLESTEROL 106 MG
SODIUM 250 MG
DIETARY FIBER 1 G

Sweet-tasting, tender trout gains a counterpoint from bread crumbs and crushed macadamia nuts. The nuts, though high in fat, are used to good advantage as a last-minute garnish; feel free to leave them out, though, if you wish.

RAINBOW TROUT

Serves 6

2 egg whites
1 cup (4 oz/125 g) Seasoned
  Bread Crumbs *(recipe on page 125)*
⅛ teaspoon freshly ground pepper
6 trout fillets, 6 oz (185 g) each,
  skin intact
1 tablespoon unsalted butter
¼ cup (2 fl oz/60 ml) fresh
  orange juice
1 tablespoon light rum
¼ cup (1½ oz/45 g) Nut Crumbs
  made with macadamias *(recipe on
  page 125),* optional
¼ cup (¼ oz/8 g) fresh basil
  leaves, finely chopped

*Nutritional Analysis
Per Serving:*

**CALORIES 324
(KILOJOULES 1,359)
PROTEIN 37 G
CARBOHYDRATES 2 G
TOTAL FAT 17 G
SATURATED FAT 4 G
CHOLESTEROL 104 MG
SODIUM 108 MG
DIETARY FIBER 0 G**

1. Preheat an oven to 400°F (200°C). Coat a 3-qt (3-l) baking pan with nonstick cooking spray.

2. In a shallow bowl, lightly beat the egg whites. In another bowl, stir together the Seasoned Bread Crumbs and pepper. Dip the trout fillets, one at a time, first in the egg whites and then in the crumb mixture and place them in the prepared pan.

3. Bake, turning once when the first side is golden brown, until the flesh is opaque throughout when pierced with a knife, 10 minutes' total cooking time. If the fillets are uneven in their thickness, be sure the thickest portions are cooked. Transfer the trout to a platter and keep warm.

4. Place the same pan over medium-high heat on the stove top and melt the butter. Add the orange juice and rum. Cook, scraping up any browned bits on the pan bottom, until slightly thickened, 1–2 minutes.

5. To serve, spoon the sauce onto individual plates and place the crispy fish fillets on top. Garnish with the Nut Crumbs, if using, and basil.

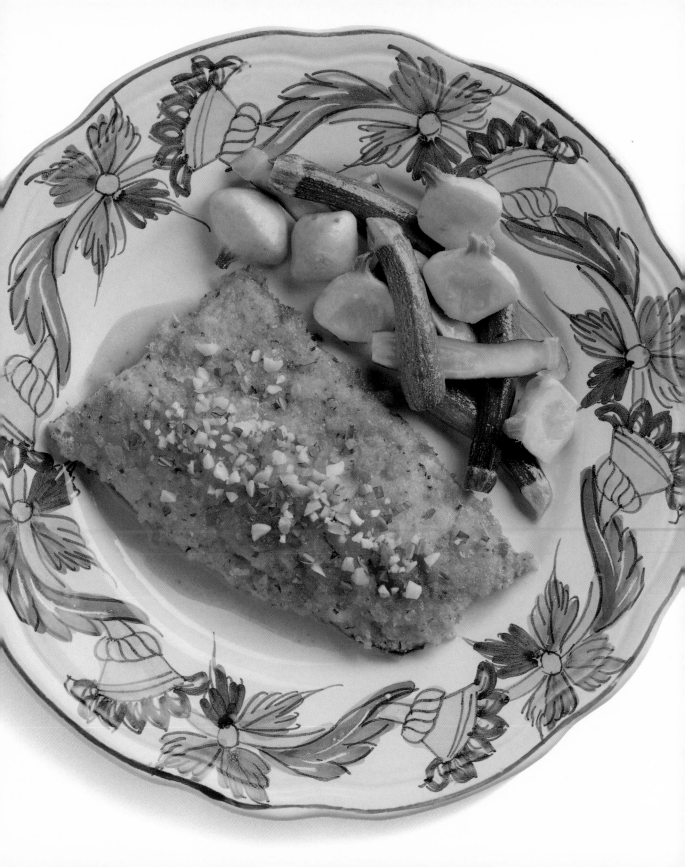

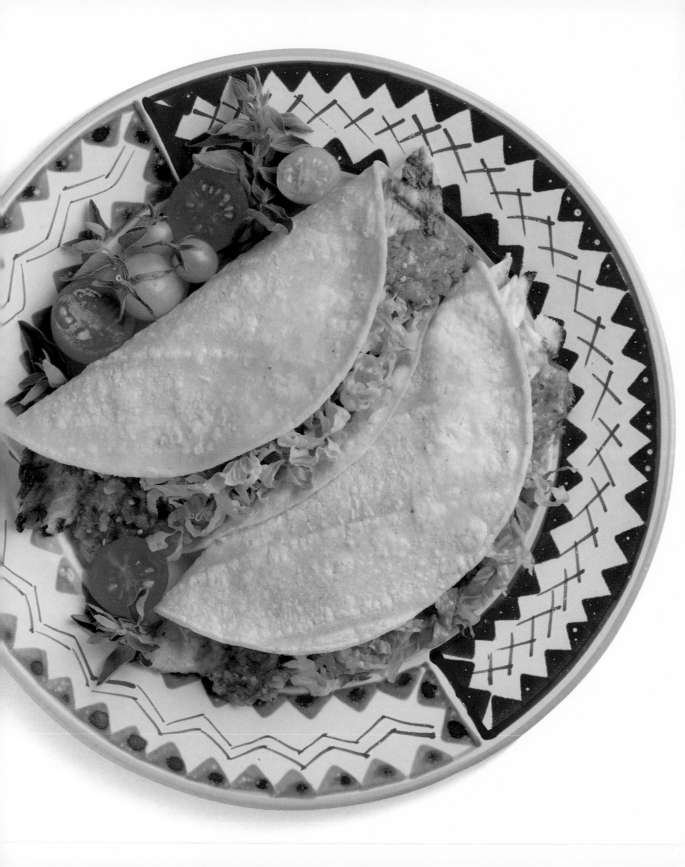

Fresh tomatillos resemble small, green tomatoes covered in brown, papery husks. They have a refreshingly tangy flavor that goes well with these fish tacos. Substitute canned tomatillos if fresh are unavailable. Mahi mahi may be used in place of snapper.

RED SNAPPER TACOS

Serves 6

1½ lb (750 g) red snapper or grouper fillets
½ cup (½ oz/15 g) fresh cilantro (fresh coriander) leaves and stems, roughly chopped
3 green (spring) onions, finely chopped
2 tablespoons olive oil
¼ cup (2 fl oz/60 ml) fresh lime juice
1 teaspoon fresh oregano
2 lb (1 kg) green tomatillos, husks intact

1 fresh chili pepper, seeded and minced, optional
12 corn tortillas, lightly dampened and wrapped in aluminum foil
1–3 teaspoons Citrus Marinade made with lime juice and tequila *(recipe on page 127)* or orange juice
4 cups (12 oz/375 g) shredded lettuce

1. Prepare a fire in a charcoal grill or preheat an oven to 400°F (200°C).
2. Place the fillets in a shallow pan. Add half of the cilantro, green onions, olive oil, lime juice and oregano. Refrigerate for 20 minutes.
3. Place the tomatillos in a hinged basket on the grill rack or on a baking tray in the oven. Cook, turning once or twice, until the skins start to bulge, 5–8 minutes. Remove and let cool.
4. Remove and discard the tomatillo husks. Quarter and place in a food processor fitted with the metal blade. Add the remaining cilantro and chili pepper, if using. Pulse to chop the tomatillos.
5. Away from the fire, coat the grill rack with nonstick cooking spray. Put the package of tortillas on the grill, near an edge, or in the oven. Remove the snapper from the marinade and discard the marinade. Place on the grill rack or in a shallow roasting pan in the oven and cook, turning once, until opaque when pierced with a knife, 4–5 minutes on each side. Cut into large chunks.
6. To assemble the tacos, remove the tortillas from the foil. Spoon an equal amount of the fish onto each tortilla and top with an equal amount of the tomatillo salsa, Citrus Marinade and lettuce.

Nutritional Analysis Per Serving:

CALORIES 313
(KILOJOULES 1,317)
PROTEIN 29 G
CARBOHYDRATES 32 G
TOTAL FAT 8 G
SATURATED FAT 1 G
CHOLESTEROL 42 MG
SODIUM 158 MG
DIETARY FIBER 3 G

Poached salmon, halibut or sea bass becomes a showstopper when graced with a dab of butter flavored with nasturtiums. First cousin to watercress, which may be substituted, the flowers provide floral sweetness and peppery bite. Wash them well before use.

POACHED SALMON WITH NASTURTIUM BUTTER

Serves 6

½ cup (4 fl oz/125 ml) fresh
   orange juice
½ cup (4 fl oz/125 ml) vodka or
   dry white wine
4 shallots, minced
¼ cup (¼ oz/8 g) nasturtium
   leaves or watercress leaves
3 salmon fillets, 8 oz (250 g)
   each, halved
⅛ teaspoon sea salt

NASTURTIUM BUTTER
2 tablespoons unsalted butter,
   at room temperature
6 nasturtium petals, minced

*Nutritional Analysis
Per Serving:*

**CALORIES 252
(KILOJOULES 1,056)
PROTEIN 23 G
CARBOHYDRATES 3 G
TOTAL FAT 11 G
SATURATED FAT 3 G
CHOLESTEROL 73 MG
SODIUM 83 MG
DIETARY FIBER 0 G**

1. Prepare the Nasturtium Butter (see below).
2. In a wide, deep frying pan large enough to hold the salmon fillets in a single layer, combine the orange juice, vodka or wine, shallots and nasturtium leaves or watercress. Bring to a boil and add the salmon fillets and salt. Reduce the heat to a gentle simmer, cover and poach until the salmon fillets are almost opaque throughout when pierced with a knife, 5–6 minutes. Uncover and cook for 2 minutes to reduce some of the liquid.
3. To serve, using a slotted spatula, transfer the fillets to individual plates. Spoon the poaching ingredients onto the plates. Slice the Nasturtium Butter into 12 pieces. Put 2 pieces on each salmon fillet.

NASTURTIUM BUTTER
1. Place the butter in a bowl. Using a wooden spoon, work the minced petals into the butter until evenly distributed.
2. Form the butter into a log and wrap in plastic wrap. Chill until serving time.

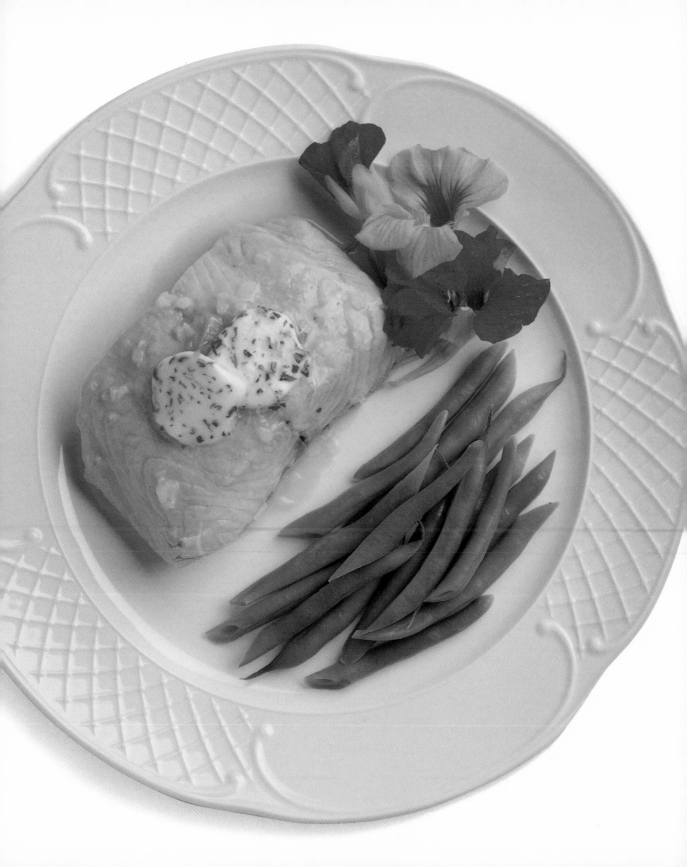

Many fish markets and food stores carry freshly cooked and frozen cooked Dungeness crab, available through midwinter. If you use these precooked crabs, follow the same method given below, lessening the steaming time to 5 minutes.

Dungeness Crab with Jalapeño Rémoulade

Serves 6

4½ cups (36 fl oz/1 l) dark beer
¾ cup (1 oz/30 g) fresh parsley stems (reserve leaves for another use)
1 teaspoon peppercorns, crushed
½ teaspoon red pepper flakes
4 bay leaves
¼ cup (2 fl oz/60 ml) fresh lemon juice
3 fresh Dungeness crabs, 6 lb (3 kg) total weight or 2 lb (1 kg) king crab legs
½ lb (250 g) French bread

Jalapeño Rémoulade
½ cup (4 fl oz/125 ml) lowfat mayonnaise
1 tablespoon whole-grain mustard
1 fresh jalapeño pepper, seeded and finely minced
½ teaspoon anchovy paste

1. In a large steamer pan, combine the beer, parsley stems, peppercorns, pepper flakes, bay leaves and lemon juice. Put the steamer rack in place. Alternatively, invert a strainer in the top of a large pot. Cover and bring to a boil. Reduce the heat to medium-low and simmer for 5 minutes.
2. Uncover and, using tongs, place the crabs on the steamer rack. Do not let the crabs touch the liquid. Re-cover and when steam begins to rise from the liquid again, steam until the crabs are bright red, about 20 minutes. If the liquid seems to be evaporating, add 2–4 cups (16–32 fl oz/500 ml–1 l) water.
3. Prepare the Jalapeño Rémoulade (see below).
4. To serve, twist off the legs and pick out the meat. Remove and discard the spongy gills. Break the body in half from front to back to reveal the meat in the sections. Accompany each serving with the bread and an equal amount of the Jalapeño Rémoulade.

Jalapeño Rémoulade
1. In a small bowl, stir together the mayonnaise, mustard, jalapeño pepper and anchovy paste. Cover and refrigerate.
2. Barely warm the sauce before serving.

Nutritional Analysis Per Serving:

Calories 256
(Kilojoules 1075)
Protein 23 g
Carbohydrates 22 g
Total Fat 8 g
Saturated Fat 2 g
Cholesterol 71 mg
Sodium 703 mg
Dietary Fiber 1 g

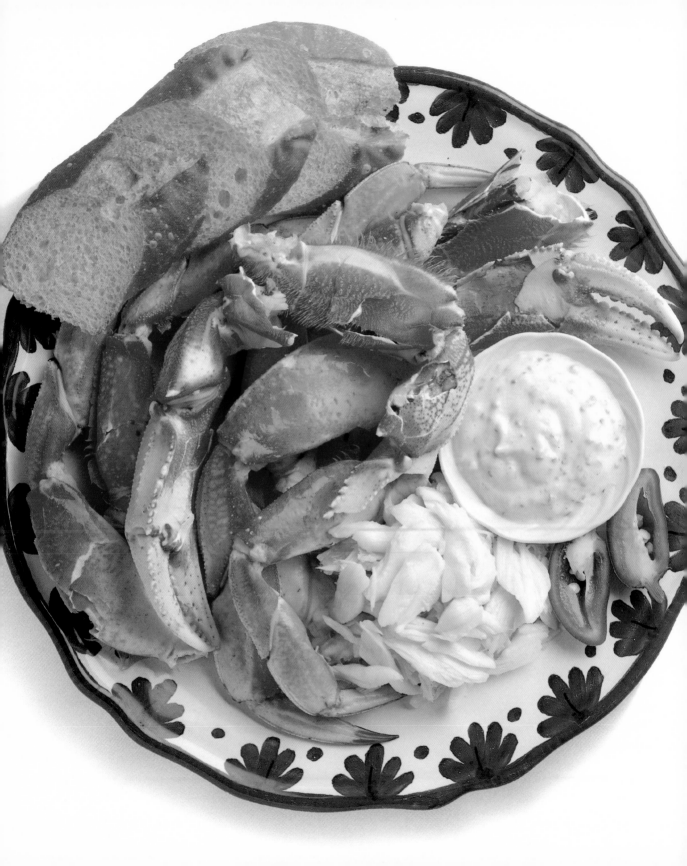

The sweet flavor of fresh squid is highlighted here by tomatoes and jalapeño chilies that have been roasted to bring out their own inherent sweetness. Peeled and deveined shrimp are a good substitute. To keep the squid from turning rubbery, take care not to overcook it.

SIMMERED SQUID

Serves 6

2½ lb (1.25 kg) ripe plum (Roma) tomatoes
1 fresh jalapeño pepper, halved and lightly seeded
1 yellow onion, peeled and cut into slices ½ inch (12 mm) wide
¼ cup (2 fl oz/60 ml) Roast Garlic Sauce *(recipe on page 126)* or 4 garlic cloves, peeled and minced and mixed with 2 tablespoons white wine vinegar

1 cup (8 fl oz/250 ml) red wine
2 cups (16 fl oz/500 ml) Vegetable Stock *(recipe on page 124)* or water
1½ lb (750 g) cleaned squid tubes and tentacles, with the tubes cut into rings ½ inch (12 mm) wide
3 tablespoons finely chopped fresh basil
3 tablespoons freshly grated Parmesan cheese

Nutritional Analysis Per Serving:

CALORIES 221
(KILOJOULES 928)
PROTEIN 21 G
CARBOHYDRATES 19 G
TOTAL FAT 4 G
SATURATED FAT 1 G
CHOLESTEROL 266 MG
SODIUM 122 MG
DIETARY FIBER 3 G

1. Preheat an oven to 400°F (200°C).
2. Arrange the tomatoes, jalapeño pepper and onion in a roasting pan. Roast until the tomatoes are soft and their skins are blistered, the jalapeño is blistered and the onion is brown, about 20 minutes.
3. In a food processor fitted with the metal blade, combine the tomatoes, jalapeño pepper, onion and Garlic Sauce. Pulse several times to form a rough purée. Spoon the mixture into a large saucepan, stir in the wine and Vegetable Stock or water and bring to a boil. Cover, reduce the heat to low and simmer for 5 minutes to blend the flavors.
4. Uncover and add the squid. Re-cover immediately and remove from the heat. Let stand for 3 minutes. The squid will cook in the trapped heat.
5. To serve, transfer to a shallow serving dish. Sprinkle with the basil and cheese.

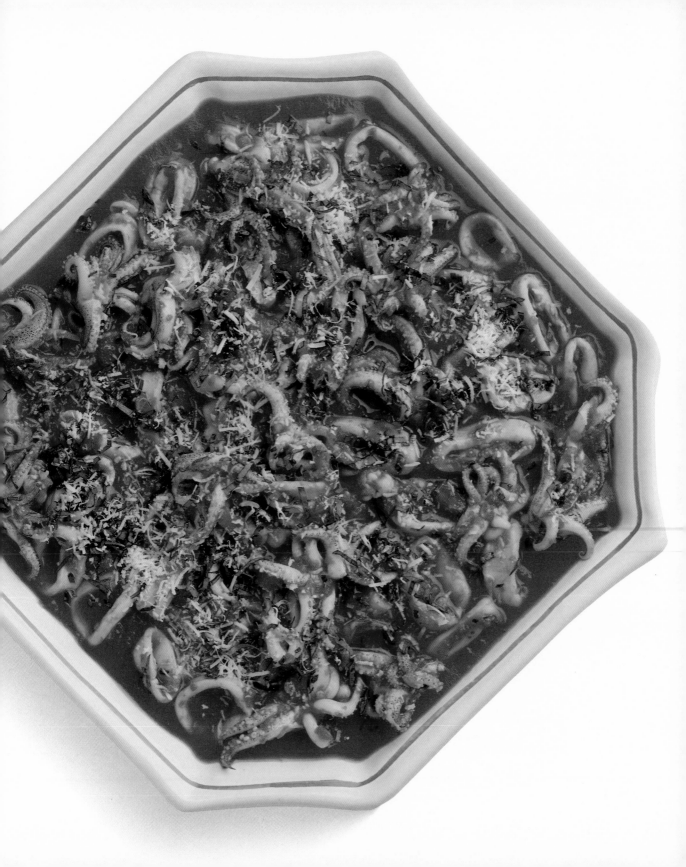

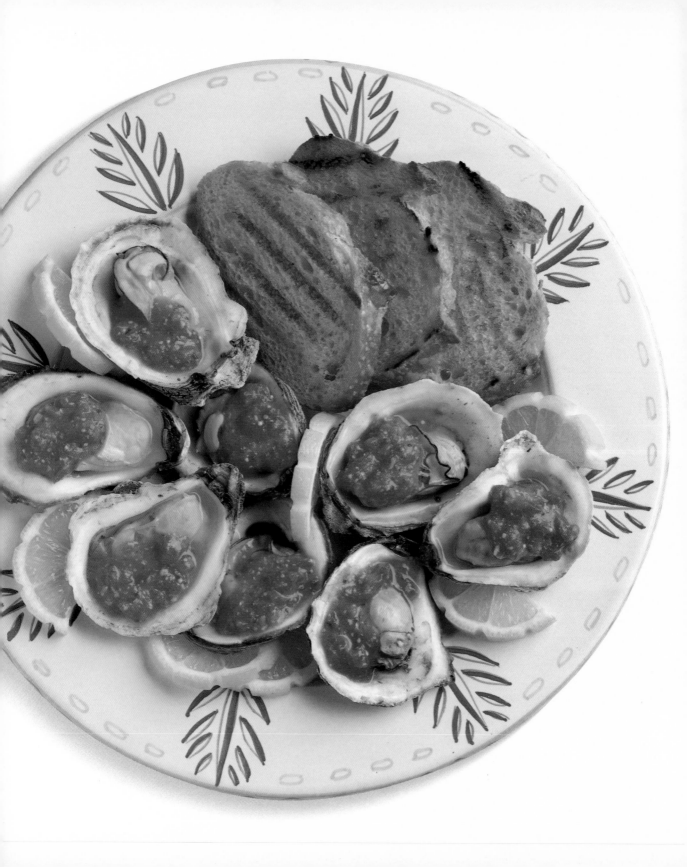

One of the simplest, most delicious ways to cook oysters, this dish makes an impressive centerpiece for a dinner party. Buy your oysters only from a quality seafood merchant and check that they are tightly closed when purchased—a sign they are alive.

Barbecued Oysters

Serves 6

1 can (14½ oz/455 g) crushed tomatoes
¼ cup Roast Garlic Sauce *(recipe on page 126)* or 4 garlic cloves, peeled and minced and mixed with 2 tablespoons white wine vinegar

1 tablespoon whole-grain mustard
1 teaspoon prepared horseradish
2 tablespoons fresh lemon juice
2 tablespoons tomato paste
4 dozen large oysters in the shell, well scrubbed

1. Prepare a fire in a charcoal grill or preheat an oven to 350°F (180°C).

2. In a bowl, stir together the tomatoes, Garlic Sauce, mustard, horseradish, lemon juice and tomato paste. Cover and refrigerate until serving.

3. Using tongs or fireproof gloves, place the oysters on the grill rack or a baking sheet, rounded-side up. Grill or bake until they open fully, about 7 minutes.

4. Again using tongs or fireproof gloves, remove each open oyster from the grill rack or baking sheet. Using a shucking or other sharp knife, cut the muscle connecting the oyster to the bottom shell. Rinse a half shell for each oyster.

5. To serve, present each oyster on the half shell topped with 1 teaspoon of the tomato mixture.

Nutritional Analysis Per Serving:

CALORIES 140
(KILOJOULES 588)
PROTEIN 11 G
CARBOHYDRATES 12 G
TOTAL FAT 5 G
SATURATED FAT 1 G
CHOLESTEROL 78 MG
SODIUM 341 MG
DIETARY FIBER 1 G

The lively flavors of tropical fruit highlight shrimp's sweet taste. Serve this vibrant dish on a summer day when mangoes are best and jumbo shrimp are in the market. Presoak wooden skewers in water for 30 minutes to prevent burning.

SKEWERED GRILLED SHRIMP WITH MANGO SALSA

Serves 6

½ cup (4 fl oz/125 ml) fresh Key lime juice
2 cups (16 fl oz/500 ml) passion fruit, orange, tangerine, pineapple or kiwifruit juice, or a mixture
½ cup (4 fl oz/125 ml) dark rum
¼ cup (⅓ oz/10 g) chopped fresh cilantro (fresh coriander)
1 tablespoon Roast Garlic Sauce *(recipe on page 126)* or 1 garlic clove, peeled and minced and mixed with 2 teaspoons white wine vinegar
red pepper flakes
salt and freshly ground pepper
1½ lb (750 g) jumbo shrimp (prawns), peeled and deveined

Nutritional Analysis Per Serving:

CALORIES 227
(KILOJOULES 952)
PROTEIN 23 G
CARBOHYDRATES 19 G
TOTAL FAT 2 G
SATURATED FAT 0 G
CHOLESTEROL 163 MG
SODIUM 162 MG
DIETARY FIBER 0 G

MANGO SALSA
1 ripe mango, peeled, pitted and cut into small pieces (1 cup/6 oz/185 g)
2 green (spring) onions, including green and white parts, finely chopped
¼ cup (⅓ oz/10 g) chopped fresh cilantro (fresh coriander)
2 tablespoons Citrus Marinade *(recipe on page 127)*

1. In a large nonreactive bowl, stir together the lime juice, fruit juice, rum, cilantro, Garlic Sauce, and red pepper flakes, salt and pepper to taste. Add the shrimp and toss to coat well. Cover and refrigerate for 2 hours.
2. Prepare the Mango Salsa (see below).
3. Prepare a fire in a charcoal grill or preheat a broiler (griller). Away from the fire, coat the grill rack with nonstick cooking spray.
4. Just before cooking, remove the shrimp from the marinade and discard the marinade. Thread the shrimp onto 6 skewers. Place the skewers on the grill or broiler rack and cook, turning once, until the shrimp turn pink, 3–4 minutes' total cooking time.
5. To serve, divide the Mango Salsa evenly among individual plates and top with a skewer of shrimp.

MANGO SALSA
1. In a small bowl, combine the mango, green onions, cilantro and Citrus Marinade. Stir to mix well.

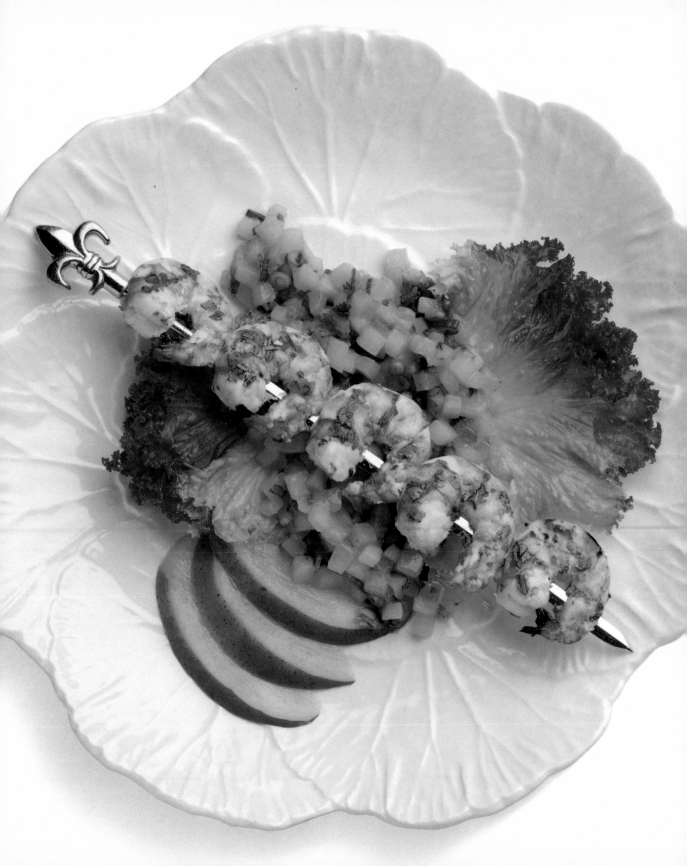

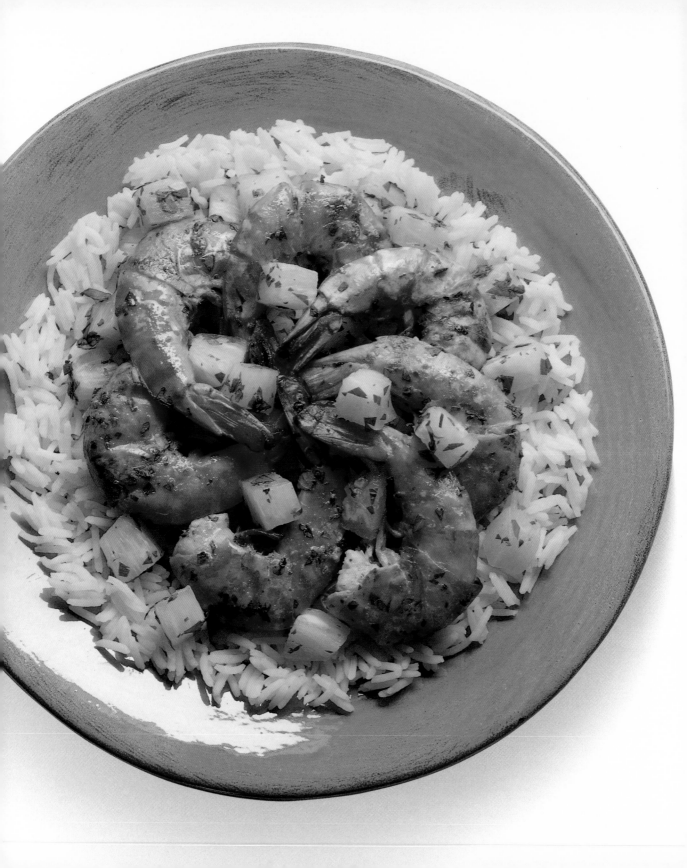

Tiger shrimp are best for this dish, because their sturdier shells help trap the seasonings, but any variety will work. Loosen the shells just enough so you can tuck in the curry mixture, keeping the legs intact to prevent the shells from falling away.

GRILLED CURRIED SHRIMP

Serves 8

2 tablespoons Roast Garlic Sauce *(recipe on page 126)* or 2 garlic cloves, peeled and minced and mixed with 1 tablespoon white wine vinegar
1 tablespoon green curry paste
¼ cup (2 fl oz/60 ml) coconut milk
½ cup (½ oz/15 g) fresh cilantro (fresh coriander) leaves, finely chopped

2 lb (1 kg) raw jumbo tiger shrimp (prawns), in their shells
4 tablespoons (2 fl oz/60 ml) fresh lemon juice
2 cups (16 fl oz/500 ml) water
1 cup (7 oz/220 g) jasmine or other fragrant rice
1 pineapple, peeled, cored and cut into ½-inch (12-mm) chunks
1 teaspoon hot chili vinegar or the liquid from bottled chilies

1. In a blender, combine the Garlic Sauce, curry paste, coconut milk and half of the cilantro until blended. Press some of the mixture in between the shrimp and their shells and place in a shallow dish. Spoon any remaining paste around the shrimp. Sprinkle with half of the lemon juice. Cover and chill for 30 minutes.
2. Place the water in a medium saucepan. Bring to a boil and add the rice. Cover the pot, turn the heat to low and simmer for 18 minutes. Turn off the heat and let sit for 5 minutes, then fluff with a fork.
3. In a large bowl, combine the pineapple, the remaining cilantro and the chili vinegar. Add enough of the remaining lemon juice to balance the sweet-tart flavors. Reserve until serving time.
4. Prepare a fire in a charcoal grill or preheat a broiler (griller).
5. Place the shrimp in a hinged basket on the grill rack or on a baking tray under the broiler (griller). Cook, turning once, until the shells are bright red, 1½–2 minutes on each side.
6. To serve, divide the rice and pineapple mixture among individual plates. Top with the grilled shrimp.

Nutritional Analysis Per Serving:

CALORIES 250
(KILOJOULES 1,049)
PROTEIN 21 G
CARBOHYDRATES 32 G
TOTAL FAT 4 G
SATURATED FAT 2 G
CHOLESTEROL 140 MG
SODIUM 155 MG
DIETARY FIBER 1 G

Complement this richly flavored dish with simple fresh, steamed asparagus.
The meat from blue crabs is slightly sweeter and less salty than that of Dungeness
crabs and is available during the summer.

CRAB & MUSHROOM CASSEROLE

Serves 6

1 cup (4 oz/125 g) freshly grated
  Parmesan cheese
¼ cup (1 oz/30 g) Seasoned Bread
  Crumbs *(recipe on page 125)*
½ cup (4 fl oz/125 ml) Vegetable
  Stock *(recipe on page 124)* or water
½ teaspoon Worcestershire sauce
2 teaspoons anisette
¾ lb (375 g) fresh oyster mushrooms

2 tablespoons unsalted butter
3 tablespoons all-purpose (plain) flour
1 cup (8 fl oz/250 ml) lowfat milk
⅛ teaspoon freshly ground pepper
hot-pepper sauce
¾ lb (375 g) crab meat, well drained,
  picked over for shell fragments and
  cartilage and flaked
2 tablespoons fresh lemon juice

*Nutritional Analysis
Per Serving:*

**CALORIES 172
(KILOJOULES 723)
PROTEIN 16 G
CARBOHYDRATES 10 G
TOTAL FAT 7 G
SATURATED FAT 4 G
CHOLESTEROL 72 MG
SODIUM 277 MG
DIETARY FIBER 1 G**

1. Preheat an oven to 350°F (180°C). Coat a 2-qt (2-l) baking
dish with nonstick cooking spray.
2. In a bowl, toss together the cheese and Seasoned Bread Crumbs.
3. In a saucepan over medium heat, combine the Vegetable Stock
or water, Worcestershire sauce, anisette and mushrooms. Bring to
a simmer and cook, uncovered, over low heat until the mushrooms
are tender, about 10 minutes. Using a slotted spoon, remove the
mushrooms. Raise the heat to medium-high and cook the liquid
until reduced by half, about 3 minutes longer.
4. While the mushrooms are cooking, in a small saucepan over
low heat, melt the butter. Whisk in the flour and cook, stirring, for
2 minutes. Then whisk in the milk, a little at a time. Cook, stirring,
until the mixture forms a thick sauce, 1–2 minutes. Add the pepper
and the hot-pepper sauce to taste.
5. Stir the stock mixture into the butter mixture. Add the reserved
mushrooms, crab meat and lemon juice and stir to mix well. Spoon
into the prepared dish. Sprinkle the cheese-crumb mixture on top.
6. Bake until browned and bubbling, about 20 minutes.

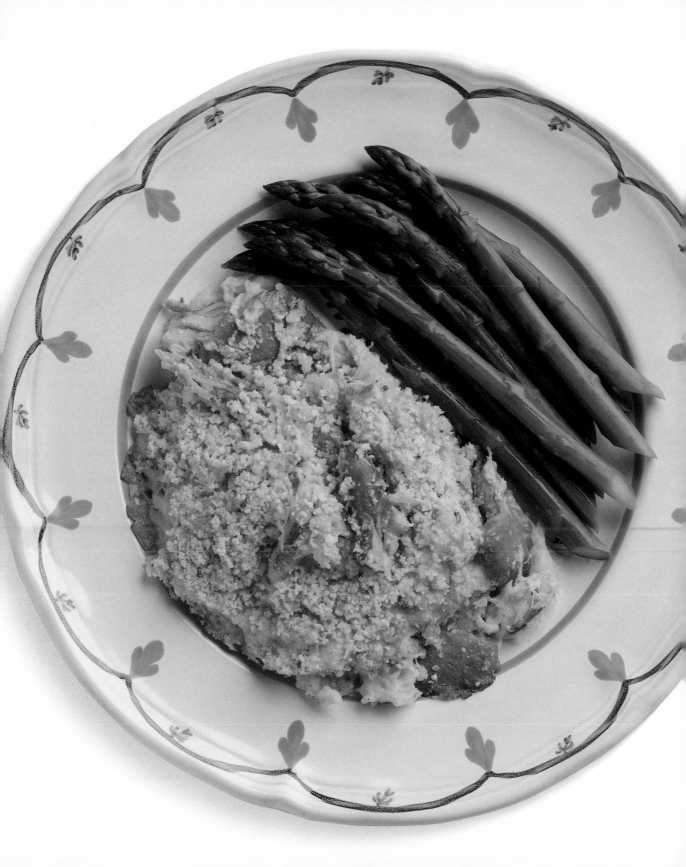

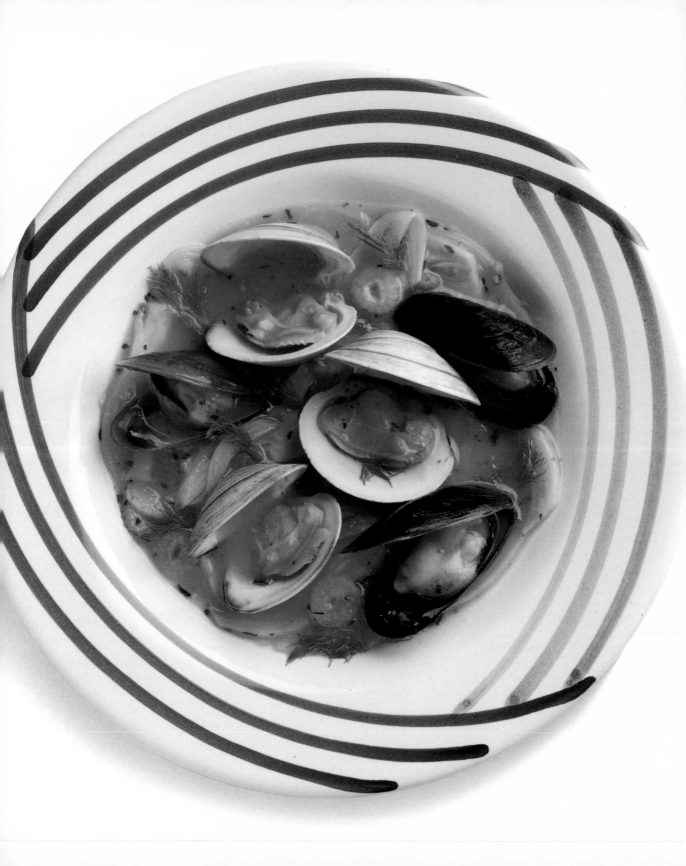

Fennel, with its crisp texture and licoricelike flavor, comes into season when mollusks are at their best. Buy mussels and clams absolutely fresh, from the most reputable merchant in your area. Discard any open shellfish.

FENNEL-FLAVORED MUSSELS & CLAMS

Serves 6

1 fennel bulb, 6 oz (185 g), with stems and fronds intact

1 tablespoon olive oil

2 tablespoons Roast Garlic Sauce *(recipe on page 126)* or 2 garlic cloves, peeled and minced and mixed with 1 tablespoon white wine vinegar

1 teaspoon herbes de Provence or ½ teaspoon each dried oregano and thyme

1 cup (8 fl oz/250 ml) dry white wine

1 cup (8 fl oz/250 ml) fresh orange juice

2 tablespoons anisette

sea salt and freshly ground pepper

18 mussels, well scrubbed and debearded if needed

18 littleneck clams, well scrubbed

1. Remove the fronds and stem from the fennel bulb and chop the fronds into ½-inch (12-mm) lengths. Set aside. Remove the tough or bruised outer leaves of the bulb and discard. Cut the bulb lengthwise into thin strips. Cut the stem into thin circles.

2. In a large, deep frying pan over medium-low heat, warm the olive oil. Add the fennel strips and stem and the Garlic Sauce and cook, stirring, until the fennel starts to soften, about 5 minutes.

3. Raise the heat to medium, add the herbes de Provence, half of the fennel fronds, the wine, orange juice, anisette and salt and pepper to taste. When the mixture is bubbling, reduce the heat to medium-low, add the mussels, cover and steam for 3 minutes. Add the clams, shake the pan, cover and steam until open, 3–4 minutes. Discard any mussels or clams that do not open.

4. To serve, using a slotted spoon, divide the fennel, mussels and clams among individual bowls. Then divide an equal amount of the cooking liquid among the bowls. Sprinkle the remaining fennel fronds over the top.

Nutritional Analysis Per Serving:

CALORIES 147
(KILOJOULES 619)
PROTEIN 9 G
CARBOHYDRATES 10 G
TOTAL FAT 4 G
SATURATED FAT 1 G
CHOLESTEROL 22 MG
SODIUM 120 MG
DIETARY FIBER 0 G

The combination of seasonings and a sauce thickened with cornstarch (cornflour) provides the richness of a classic *coquilles St. Jacques*, with far less fat. Large sea scallops make a beautiful presentation, but little bay scallops may also be used.

Sherried Sea Scallops

Serves 6

2 tablespoons unsalted butter

8 shallots, finely minced

1 tablespoon chopped fresh tarragon

1 cup (8 fl oz/250 ml) Vegetable Stock *(recipe on page 124)* or water

2 lb (1 kg) sea scallops

⅛ teaspoon salt

⅛ teaspoon white pepper

⅓ cup (3 fl oz/80 ml) dry sherry

1 cup (8 fl oz/250 ml) lowfat milk

2 tablespoons cornstarch (cornflour)

2 tablespoons minced fresh basil leaves

1. In a large frying pan over medium-low heat, melt the butter. Add the shallots and tarragon and sauté, stirring, until soft and fragrant, 2–3 minutes.

2. Add the Vegetable Stock and simmer, uncovered, for 5 minutes. Add the scallops, salt and pepper and cook, turning once, until the scallops are opaque and firm to the touch, 1–2 minutes on each side; do not overcook. Using a slotted spoon, transfer the scallops to a warmed plate, cover and keep warm.

3. Cook the liquid remaining in the frying pan, uncovered, over medium-high heat until reduced by half, about 5 minutes. In a small bowl, stir together the sherry and milk and then whisk in the cornstarch. Add to the frying pan and continue to simmer, uncovered, stirring occasionally, until the sauce thickens and is fragrant, 2–3 minutes.

4. To serve, divide the scallops equally among individual plates. Spoon the sauce evenly over the scallops. Sprinkle with the basil.

Nutritional Analysis Per Serving:

CALORIES 227

(KILOJOULES 953)

PROTEIN 27 G

CARBOHYDRATES 12 G

TOTAL FAT 5 G

SATURATED FAT 3 G

CHOLESTEROL 62 MG

SODIUM 316 MG

DIETARY FIBER 0 G

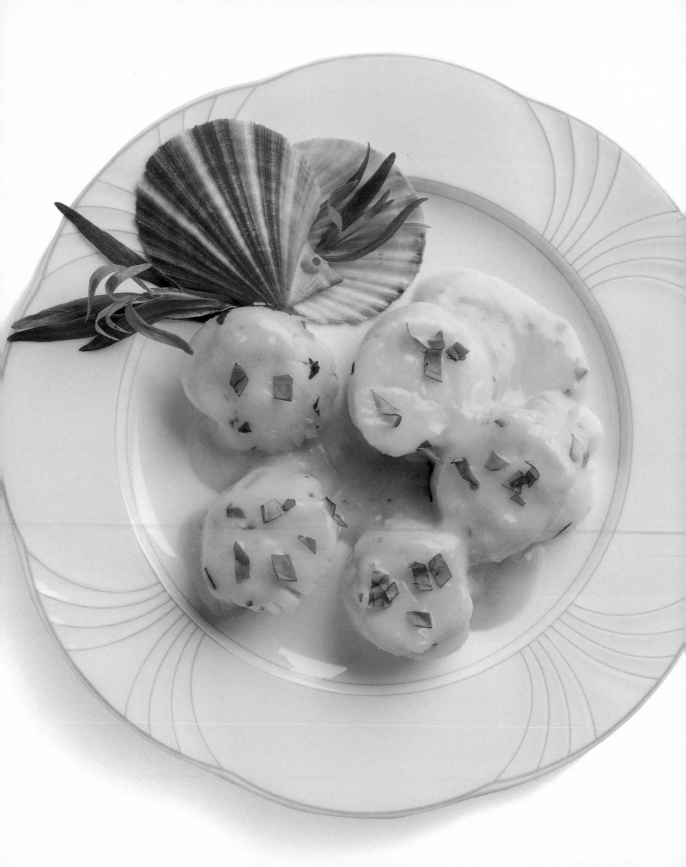

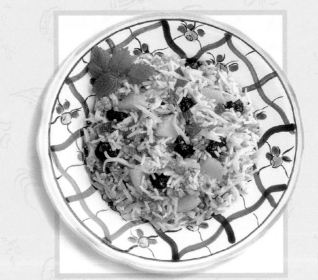

PASTA, GRAINS & BEANS

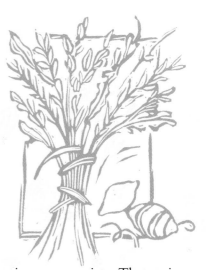

$\mathscr{P}$olenta, couscous, red lentils, lasagna, bulgur pilaf: Looking through the recipes in this chapter can seem like an tour of the world's most rustic cuisines. Indeed, such time-honored food offers a lesson in healthy eating that many cooks are only just beginning to appreciate: That main dish recipes featuring grains, pasta and beans number among the wisest, most satisfying choices for today's health-conscious cook. Some recipes use those featured ingredients as a way to extend a relatively small amount of animal protein. Still others are strictly vegetarian, combining two or more sources of vegetable protein to provide all the essential amino acids necessary for good nutrition. Virtually all are low in fat, saturated fat and cholesterol. Try these recipes as a change of pace from your usual main dish meat, poultry or seafood. Several times a week let pasta, grains and beans move from the side of your dinner plate to center stage, where they rightly belong. As an added benefit, these well-balanced recipes easily become one-dish meals, simplifying cooking for the busy food preparer.

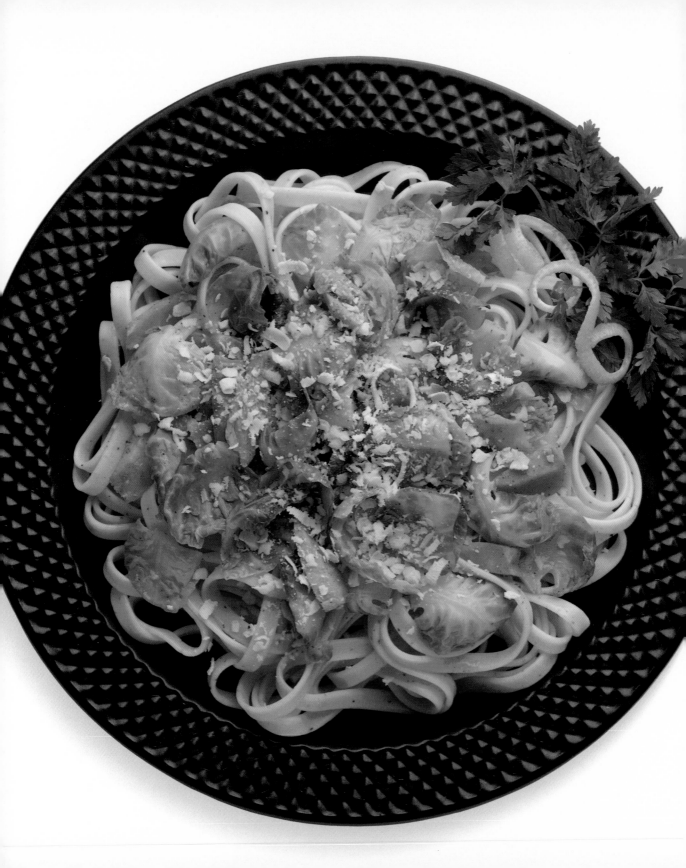

This recipe uses sapsago, a pungent, hard, light-green cheese from Switzerland, with less than 10 percent fat. If you can't find it, substitute an equal amount of feta, rinsed to remove excess salt. If lemon-pepper is unavailable, use regular fettuccine.

LEMON–BLACK PEPPER PASTA

Serves 6

1 cup (8 fl oz/250 ml) Chicken Stock
  (recipe on page 124)
2 oz (60 g) smoked turkey, slivered
¼ teaspoon five-spice powder
¾ lb (375 g) Brussels sprouts
1 lb (500 g) dried lemon–black pepper fettuccine
2 tablespoons grated sapsago cheese

1. Fill a large pot three-fourths full of water, place over high heat and bring to a boil.
2. Meanwhile, in a deep frying pan over medium heat, combine the Chicken Stock, turkey, five-spice powder and Brussels sprouts. Bring to a simmer and cook until the stock begins to thicken, the turkey is heated through and the sprout leaves have turned deeper green, 8–10 minutes.
3. While the sauce is simmering, add the pasta to the boiling water and cook according to package directions or until al dente, 8–10 minutes.
4. To serve, drain the pasta and place in a shallow serving bowl. Add the sauce and top with the cheese.

Nutritional Analysis Per Serving:

CALORIES 338
(KILOJOULES 1,419)
PROTEIN 15 G
CARBOHYDRATES 60 G
TOTAL FAT 4 G
SATURATED FAT 1 G
CHOLESTEROL 79 MG
SODIUM 211 MG
DIETARY FIBER 5 G

Sweet and robust Roast Garlic Sauce is an ideal complement to cooked pasta.
Leave the Parmesan cheese out if you want to cut down on the fat.
Serve with yellow and red cherry tomatoes for a colorful meal.

Spaghetti with Roast Garlic Sauce

Serves 6

1 lb (500 g) dried spaghetti
1 cup (8 fl oz/250 ml) Roast
  Garlic Sauce, at room
  temperature *(recipe on page 126)*

½ cup (2 oz/60 g) Nut Crumbs made
  with walnuts *(recipe on page 125)*
½ cup (2 oz/60 g) freshly grated
  Parmesan cheese, optional

1. Fill a large pot three-fourths full of water, place over high
heat and bring to a boil. Add the pasta and cook according to
package directions or until al dente, 8–10 minutes.
2. To serve, drain the pasta and place in a shallow serving
bowl. Spoon on the Garlic Sauce and toss to mix well. Top
with the Nut Crumbs and cheese, if using.

*Nutritional Analysis
Per Serving:*

**CALORIES 475
(KILOJOULES 1,994)
PROTEIN 16 G
CARBOHYDRATES 68 G
TOTAL FAT 17 G
SATURATED FAT 2 G
CHOLESTEROL 0 MG
SODIUM 10 MG
DIETARY FIBER 3 G**

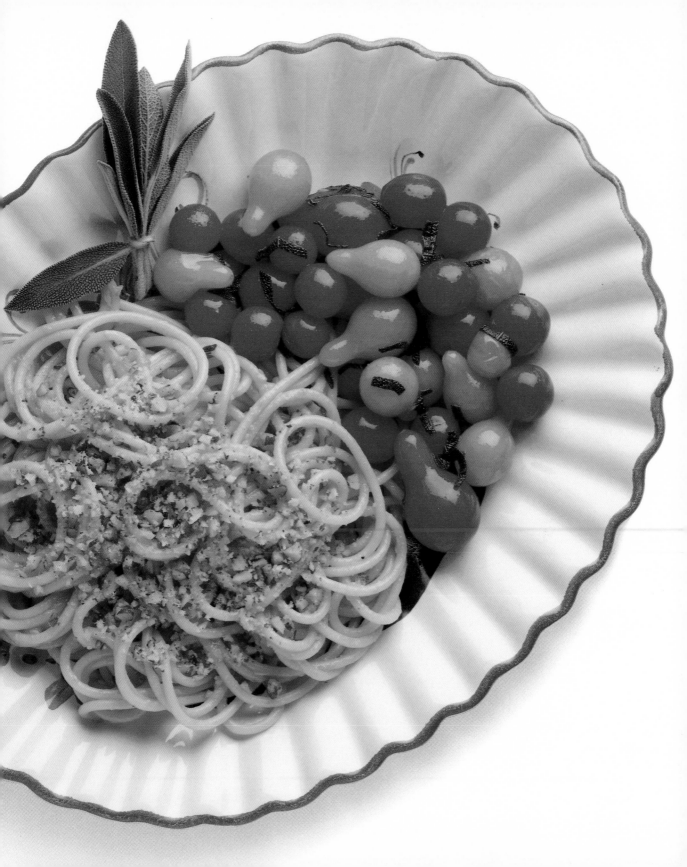

Charcoal-grilling the vegetables seals in their juices and intensifies their natural flavors, yielding excellent results with little added fat or salt. You can enhance the flavor further by cooking over fragrant woods such as mesquite, hickory or pecan.

Wild Mushroom Fettuccine

Serves 6

½ lb (250 g) firm tofu, in one piece
1 cup (8 fl oz/250 ml) Vegetable
  Stock *(recipe on page 124)* or water
1 tablespoon miso
2 tablespoons Roast Garlic Sauce
  (recipe on page 126) or 2 garlic cloves,
  peeled and minced and mixed with
  1 tablespoon white wine vinegar
1 tablespoon dry sherry
1 tablespoon fresh lemon juice

2 fresh portobello mushrooms, each 4 inches
  (10 cm) in diameter and 8 oz (250 g), cut
  into thick slices
2 red bell peppers (capsicums), seeded, deribbed
  and cut into long strips, each about ¼ inch
  (6 mm) wide
¼ cup (¼ oz/8 g) fresh flat-leaf (Italian)
  parsley leaves, roughly chopped
2 tablespoons olive oil
1 lb (500 g) fresh or dried fettuccine

*Nutritional Analysis
Per Serving:*

**Calories 353
(Kilojoules 1,484)
Protein 17 g
Carbohydrates 50 g
Total Fat 11 g
Saturated Fat 1 g
Cholesterol 89 mg
Sodium 136 mg
Dietary Fiber 1 g**

1. Place the tofu on several layers of paper towels on the counter and then top with several more layers of towels. Put a heavy plate on top and let the tofu drain for a couple of hours, to make it firm enough for grilling. Cut the tofu into 1-inch (2.5-cm) cubes.
2. In a wide, shallow dish, stir together the Vegetable Stock or water, miso, Garlic Sauce, sherry, lemon juice, mushrooms, peppers and parsley; toss to coat evenly. Let stand for 15–30 minutes.
3. Meanwhile, prepare a fire in a charcoal grill or preheat a broiler (griller). When the coals are medium-hot, brush the mushrooms, peppers and tofu with the olive oil. Place the mushrooms and peppers in a hinged grilling basket on the grill rack or on a baking tray under the broiler (griller). Cook, turning once or twice, until the vegetables are soft, about 10 minutes. Add the tofu and continue to cook until everything is browned, 2–3 minutes longer.
4. While the vegetables are cooking, put the remaining stock mixture in a frying pan over medium heat and bring to a simmer. Cook until reduced by half, about 5 minutes.

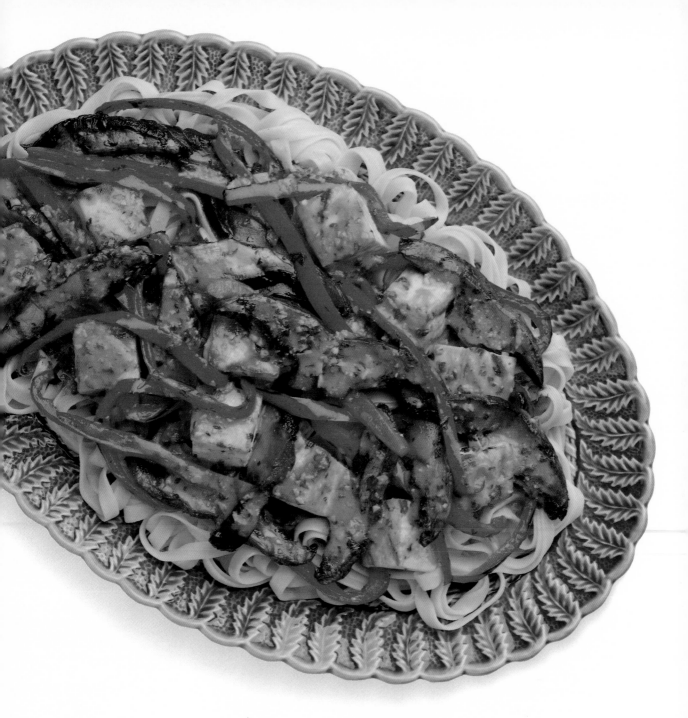

5. Fill a large pot three-fourths full with water, place over high heat and bring to a boil. Add the fettuccine and cook according to package directions or until al dente, 1–2 minutes for fresh and 8–10 minutes for dried.
6. To serve, drain the pasta and place in a shallow serving bowl. Top with the vegetables and drizzle with the reduced stock mixture.

Choose smaller, fancy-grade yellow squash or zucchini, which have finer textures and fewer large seeds. You can make the paste of olives, anchovies and sun-dried tomatoes in a food processor or, for a coarser texture, with a mortar and pestle.

Summer Squash & Bow Tie Pasta

Serves 6

1 lb (500 g) dried bow tie pasta

1 lb (500 g) yellow summer squash, thinly sliced

1 can (8 oz/250 g) pitted black olives, drained and rinsed to remove excess salt

¼ cup (2 oz/60 g) sun-dried tomatoes packed in oil, finely shredded

1 can (2 oz/60 g) anchovy fillets packed in oil, well drained and rinsed

2 tablespoons oil from sun-dried tomatoes and anchovies

¼ cup (1 oz/30 g) freshly grated Parmesan cheese, plus 2 tablespoons freshly grated Parmesan cheese, optional

¼ cup (¼ oz/7 g) fresh basil leaves, roughly chopped

¼ teaspoon freshly ground pepper

Nutritional Analysis Per Serving:

CALORIES 466

(KILOJOULES 1,956)

PROTEIN 15 G

CARBOHYDRATES 65 G

TOTAL FAT 17 G

SATURATED FAT 3 G

CHOLESTEROL 7 MG

SODIUM 610 MG

DIETARY FIBER 4 G

1. Fill a large pot three-fourths full of water, place over high heat and bring to a boil. Add the pasta and cook according to package directions or until al dente, 8–10 minutes.

2. Once the pasta is in the water, scoop out a ladleful of the hot pasta water and place it in a frying pan over high heat. Bring to a boil and add the squash. Reduce the heat to medium, cover and simmer until tender-crisp, 1–2 minutes. Drain and keep warm.

3. Meanwhile, in a food processor fitted with the metal blade, combine the olives, tomatoes, anchovies and oil and pulse just until the ingredients are finely chopped and combined. Stir in the ¼ cup (1 oz/30 g) Parmesan cheese.

4. To serve, drain the pasta and place in a shallow serving bowl. Add the olive mixture and toss to mix well. Add the squash and toss again. Sprinkle with the chopped basil and pepper. Pass the grated Parmesan cheese, if using.

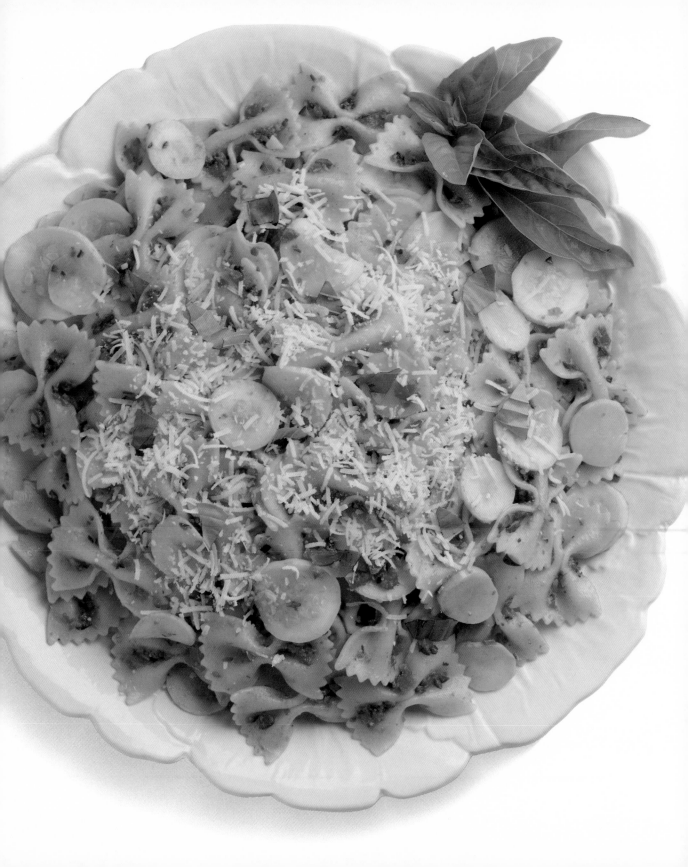

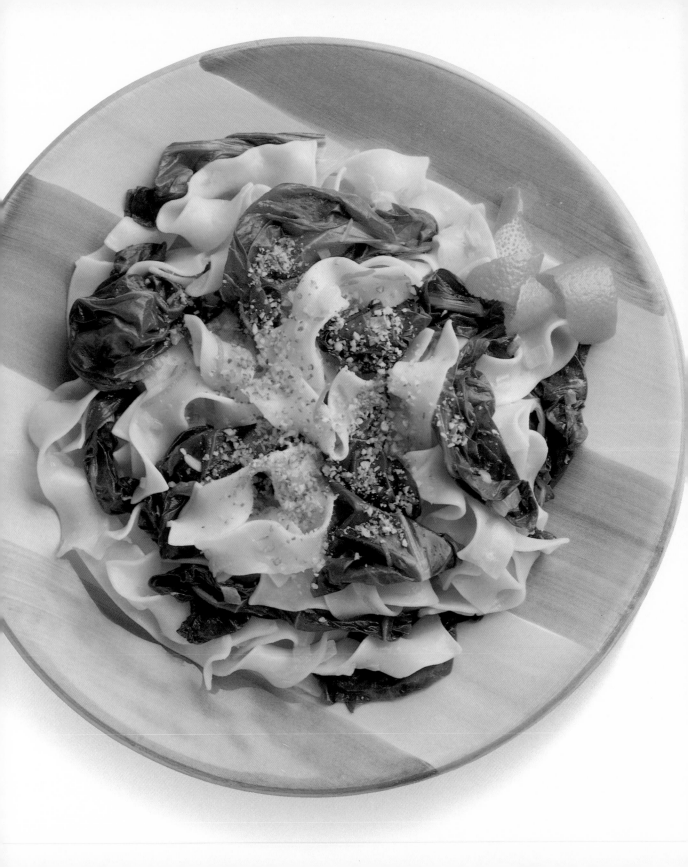

Delicate new greens or tiny interior leaves will sauté to tender crispness in minutes. If you opt for chard, use the green variety; red chard will color the sauce. Buttermilk yields a rich, smooth sauce with minimal fat.

Noodles & Sautéed Swiss Chard

Serves 6

1 tablespoon olive oil
1 large white onion, finely chopped
2 tablespoons grated orange zest
1 tablespoon triple sec
1 lb (500 g) eggless noodles
¼ cup (2 fl oz/60 ml) lowfat
  buttermilk
salt and freshly ground pepper

2 lbs (1 kg) baby Swiss chard (silverbeet)
  or turnip, mustard or collard greens,
  4–8 inches (10–20 cm) long, washed
  and stemmed
3 tablespoons Nut Crumbs made with
  pecans *(recipe on page 125)*
zest from ½ orange, optional

1. In a large frying pan, heat the olive oil. Add the onion and sauté over medium-low heat until fragrant and translucent, 10 minutes. Stir in the orange zest and triple sec and sauté 1 minute longer.
2. Fill a large pot three-fourths full of water, place over high heat and bring to a boil. Add the noodles and cook according to package directions or until al dente, 5–8 minutes.
3. While the noodles are cooking, add the buttermilk, salt and pepper to taste and the onion mixture to the frying pan and cook for 2 minutes. Add the chard or other greens, cover and turn off the heat. Let the chard barely wilt, 3–5 minutes.
4. To serve, drain the noodles and divide among individual plates. Add the chard mixture and toss to mix well. Sprinkle with the Nut Crumbs. Garnish with the zest, if using.

Nutritional Analysis Per Serving:

**Calories 365
(Kilojoules 1,531)
Protein 14 g
Carbohydrates 64 g
Total Fat 7 g
Saturated Fat 1 g
Cholesterol 0 mg
Sodium 328 mg
Dietary Fiber 3 g**

Lowfat cottage cheese contributes creamy richness without the higher fat of traditional lasagna ingredients. If possible, refrigerate the assembled casserole for several hours before baking to allow the flavors to marry.

SPINACH & HERB LASAGNA

Serves 6

1 cup (1 oz/30 g) mixed fresh herbs such as flat-leaf (Italian) parsley, mint, basil, sorrel and oregano, in any combination

2 cups (1 lb/500 g) lowfat cottage cheese

2 oz (60 g) sharp pecorino romano cheese, grated

3 tablespoons Roast Garlic Sauce *(recipe on page 126)* or 3 garlic cloves, peeled and minced and mixed with 1½ tablespoons white wine vinegar

2 eggs, lightly beaten

4 cups (4 oz/125 g) small spinach leaves or Swiss chard (silverbeet), stemmed, carefully washed and fully dried

2 cups (16 fl oz/500 ml) Quick Tomato Sauce *(recipe on page 126)*

1 can (8 fl oz/250 ml) tomato paste

1 lb (500 g) fresh or dried lasagna noodles

Nutritional Analysis Per Serving:

CALORIES 497
(KILOJOULES 2,085)
PROTEIN 28 G
CARBOHYDRATES 75 G
TOTAL FAT 10 G
SATURATED FAT 2 G
CHOLESTEROL 87 MG
SODIUM 816 MG
DIETARY FIBER 5 G

1. Preheat an oven to 350°F (180°C). Coat an 8-by-10-by-2-inch (20-by-25-by-5-cm) baking dish with nonstick cooking spray.

2. Fill a large pot three-fourths full of water, place over high heat and bring to a boil.

3. While the water is coming to a boil, in a bowl, combine the herbs, cottage cheese, half of the pecorino romano cheese, the Garlic Sauce and eggs. Stir to mix well. Stir the spinach into this mixture. In a separate bowl, stir together the Quick Tomato Sauce and tomato paste.

4. Add the noodles to the boiling water and cook according to package directions or until al dente, 4–5 minutes for fresh and 12–15 minutes for dried. Drain, being careful not to tear the noodles. Lay the noodles flat in a single layer on towels.

5. To assemble the dish, spoon a little of the Quick Tomato Sauce mixture into the bottom of the prepared baking dish. Cover the sauce with a layer of noodles overlapping the edges slightly. Spoon a thin layer of the cheese filling over the noodles and top with a little more of the Quick Tomato Sauce mixture. Repeat the layers until all the noodles, cheese filling and Quick Tomato Sauce mixture are used, ending with the sauce. Sprinkle the remaining pecorino romano cheese evenly over the top.

6. Bake until the lasagna is bubbling and the edges are brown, about 45 minutes.

7. To serve, remove from the oven and let sit 5 minutes before scooping onto individual plates.

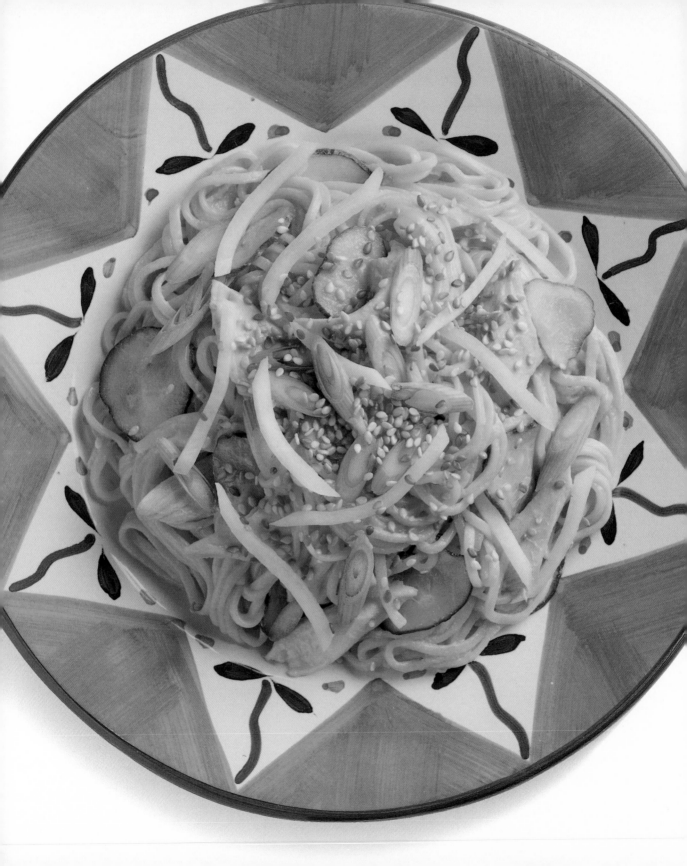

Soba noodles, made from buckwheat and wheat flour, add wonderful flavor to this carbohydrate-rich dish; look for them in Asian or natural-food shops. Pickling cucumbers are widely available most of the summer. If you use a large cucumber, peel and seed it.

CHICKEN & CUCUMBERS ON SESAME NOODLES

Serves 6

¼ cup (1 oz/30 g) sesame seeds
2 tablespoons low-sodium soy sauce
1 tablespoon rice wine vinegar
1 tablespoon Flavored Sesame Oil
  (recipe on page 127)
1 tablespoon Roast Garlic Sauce
  (recipe on page 126) or 1 garlic clove,
  peeled and minced and mixed with
  2 teaspoons white wine vinegar
2 tablespoons tahini, well stirred,
  or peanut butter

½ teaspoon sea salt
¾ lb (375 g) soba noodles
1½ cups (9 oz/280 g) shredded skinned
  cooked chicken meat
3 pickling cucumbers, 8 oz (250 g)
  total weight, thinly sliced
6 green (spring) onions, thinly sliced
1 piece daikon, 2 inches (5 cm) long,
  thinly sliced, optional

1. To toast the sesame seeds, place them in a small frying pan over high heat and toast, shaking the pan constantly, until the seeds are fragrant and golden brown, about 30 seconds.
2. Fill a large pot three-fourths full of water and place over high heat. Bring to a boil.
3. While the water is coming to a boil, combine the soy sauce, rice wine vinegar, Flavored Sesame Oil, Garlic Sauce, tahini and salt in a bowl and stir until smooth.
4. Add the noodles to the boiling water and cook according to package directions or until al dente, 5–8 minutes. Drain and place in a large serving bowl.
5. Pour the sauce over the warm noodles and toss gently to coat the noodles completely. Add the chicken and cucumbers and toss again to distribute evenly.
6. To serve, garnish the noodles with green onions, daikon, if using, and sesame seeds. Serve warm, at room temperature or chilled.

Nutritional Analysis Per Serving:

CALORIES 380
(KILOJOULES 1,597)
PROTEIN 24 G
CARBOHYDRATES 50 G
TOTAL FAT 12 G
SATURATED FAT 2 G
CHOLESTEROL 38 MG
SODIUM 775 MG
DIETARY FIBER 2 G

Italy's popular cornmeal mush provides an ideal backdrop for such hearty flavors and textures as woodsy mushrooms and fragrant croutons. If you like, chill the polenta until firm, then slice it into slabs and broil or grill until crisp and golden.

POLENTA & MUSHROOMS

Serves 6

6 cups (48 fl oz/1.5 l) Vegetable Stock or Chicken Stock *(recipes on page 124)*

¼ teaspoon sea salt

2 cups (10 oz/210 g) water-ground coarse yellow cornmeal

1 tablespoon olive oil

1 large or 2 medium leeks, white part only, carefully washed and thinly sliced

2 lb (1 kg) mixed fresh mushrooms such as cremini, shiitake, oyster, porcini and portobello, thickly sliced

1 celeriac, (8 oz/250 g) peeled and diced, or 2 celery stalks, diced

2 tablespoons Roast Garlic Sauce *(recipe on page 126)* or 2 garlic cloves, peeled and minced and mixed with 1 tablespoon white wine vinegar

½ cup (4 fl oz/125 ml) dry white wine

1 teaspoon herbes de Provence or ½ teaspoon each dried oregano and thyme

1 cup (1½ oz/45 g) Seasoned Croutons *(recipe on page 125)*

Nutritional Analysis Per Serving:

CALORIES 314

(KILOJOULES 1,318)

PROTEIN 9 G

CARBOHYDRATES 57 G

TOTAL FAT 5 G

SATURATED FAT 1 G

CHOLESTEROL 0 MG

SODIUM 145 MG

DIETARY FIBER 6 G

1. To make the polenta, in a large saucepan, bring the Vegetable or Chicken Stock and salt to a boil. Slowly pour the cornmeal in a steady stream through your fingers into the boiling stock. (This method will keep the polenta from lumping.) Reduce the heat to medium-low and cook, stirring occasionally, for 25 minutes.

2. Meanwhile, in a large frying pan over medium heat, warm the olive oil. Add the leek and sauté, stirring, until softened, about 5 minutes. Add the mushrooms and celery root; toss and cook until the mushrooms start to release their liquid, about 5 minutes.

3. Add the Garlic Sauce, wine and dried herbs to the mushrooms. Stir to mix well and continue to cook over low heat, stirring occasionally, until the sauce begins to thicken, about 20 minutes.

4. To serve, spoon the polenta into individual soup plates. Top with the mushroom mixture and Seasoned Croutons.

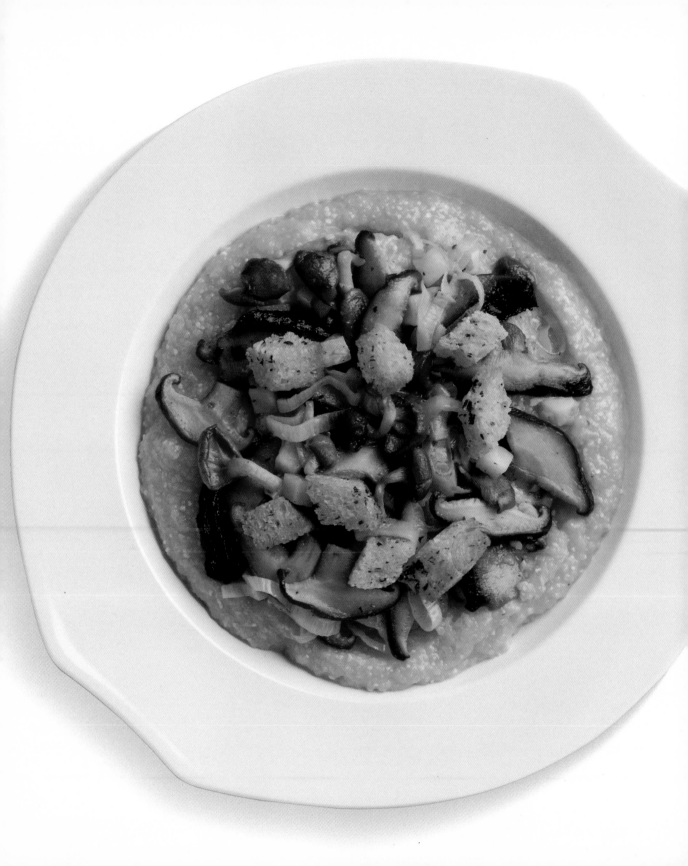

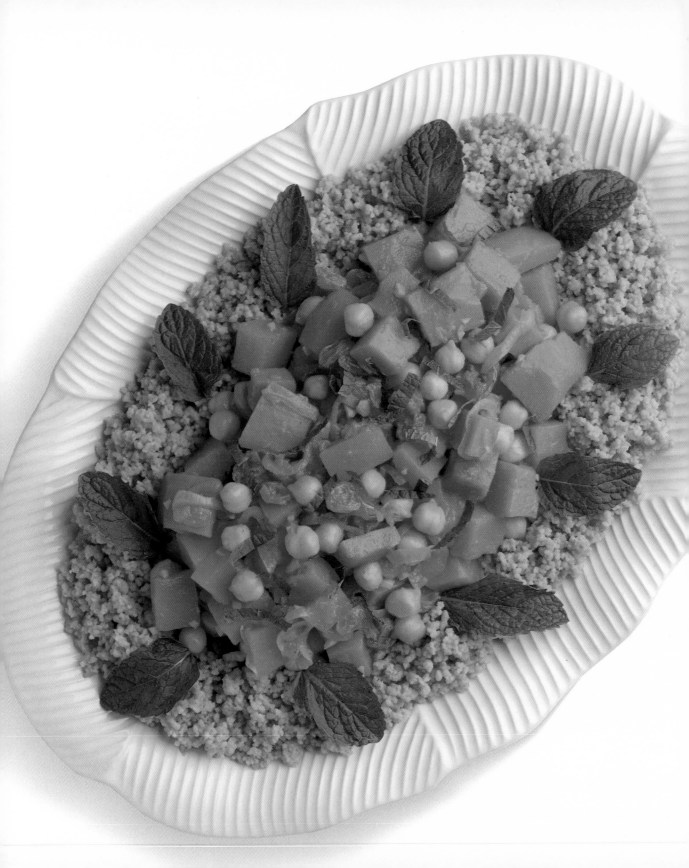

Whole-wheat couscous, available in natural-food stores, offers the full nutritional value of a whole grain and takes just a bit longer to cook than regular instant couscous. Sweet potatoes, parsnips and rutabagas (swedes) can be substituted for the squash.

WHOLE-WHEAT COUSCOUS

Serves 6

2 tablespoons unsalted butter

1 large yellow onion, thinly sliced

2 garlic cloves, peeled and chopped

2 teaspoons ground cumin

½ teaspoon coriander seeds

1 butternut squash, 3 lb (1.5 kg),
   peeled, seeded and cut into
   1-inch (2.5-cm) cubes

1 teaspoon ground ginger

⅛ teaspoon powdered saffron,
   optional

3 cups (24 fl oz/750 ml) Vegetable
   Stock *(recipe on page 124)* or water

½ cup (3 oz/90 g) golden raisins

⅛ teaspoon salt

1 can (16 oz/500 g) chick-peas
   (garbanzo beans), drained

1/16 teaspoon ground dried chili

1 cup (8 oz/250 g) whole-wheat couscous

¼ cup (¼ oz/8 g) fresh mint leaves,
   roughly chopped

3 tablespoons Nut Crumbs made with
   almonds *(recipe on page 125),* optional

1. In a large, heavy pot over medium-low heat, melt the butter. Add the onion and sauté until fragrant and translucent, about 5 minutes. Add the garlic, cumin, coriander seeds, squash, ginger, saffron, if using, and 1 cup (8 fl oz/250 ml) of the Vegetable Stock or water. Bring to a simmer, cover and simmer until the squash is tender when pierced with a fork, about 30 minutes.

2. Stir in the raisins, salt, chick-peas and ground chili. Cook for 10 minutes longer.

3. While the squash is cooking, in a saucepan, bring the remaining 2 cups (16 fl oz/500 ml) Vegetable Stock or water to a boil. Stir in the couscous and reduce the heat to low. Cover and cook the couscous for 5 minutes, then turn off the heat and let the grains stand, covered, for 5 minutes. Set aside until serving.

4. To serve, place the couscous on a platter. Top with the squash mixture. Sprinkle with the mint and Nut Crumbs, if using.

*Nutritional Analysis
Per Serving:*

**CALORIES 345
(KILOJOULES 1,447)
PROTEIN 10 G
CARBOHYDRATES 68 G
TOTAL FAT 6 G
SATURATED FAT 3 G
CHOLESTEROL 10 MG
SODIUM 143 MG
DIETARY FIBER 3 G**

Buy coarse-grind bulgur or a bulgur–soy grits mixture, available in natural-food stores; prepacked bulgur for tabbouleh has too fine a texture for this rustic dish. If you like, stir in 1 tablespoon miso or grated cheese before serving.

Bulgur Pilaf

Serves 4

2 cups (16 fl oz/500 ml) Vegetable Stock *(recipe on page 124)* or water
3 green (spring) onions or 1 leek, white part only, thinly sliced
2 tablespoons peeled and grated fresh ginger
grated zest of 1 large orange

2 cups (12 oz/375 g) bulgur
¼ cup (1½ oz/45 g) dried currants
¼ cup (¼ oz/8 g) fresh flat-leaf (Italian) parsley leaves, roughly chopped
¼ teaspoon sea salt, optional
2 teaspoons raspberry vinegar
¼ cup (1 oz/30 g) Nut Crumbs made with pecans *(recipe on page 125)*

1. In a large frying pan over medium heat, bring half of the Vegetable Stock or water to a simmer. Add the onions or leek, ginger and half of the orange zest. Simmer until the mixture is fragrant and the onions are softened, about 5 minutes.
2. Stir in the bulgur, currants, parsley, the remaining Vegetable Stock and the salt, if using. Cover and simmer until the bulgur has absorbed the liquid, about 10 minutes.
3. Turn off the heat and stir in the remaining orange zest. Let stand, covered, for 5 minutes.
4. To serve, transfer to a serving bowl. Sprinkle with the raspberry vinegar and Nut Crumbs.

Nutritional Analysis Per Serving:

**Calories 327
(Kilojoules 1,374)
Protein 10 g
Carbohydrates 64 g
Total Fat 6 g
Saturated Fat 1 g
Cholesterol 0 mg
Sodium 22 mg
Dietary Fiber 14 g**

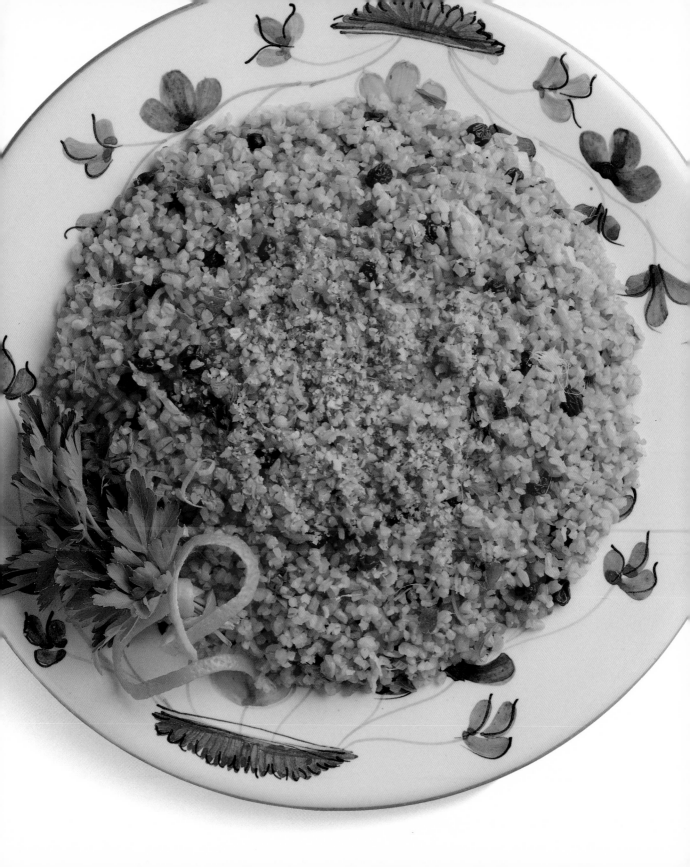

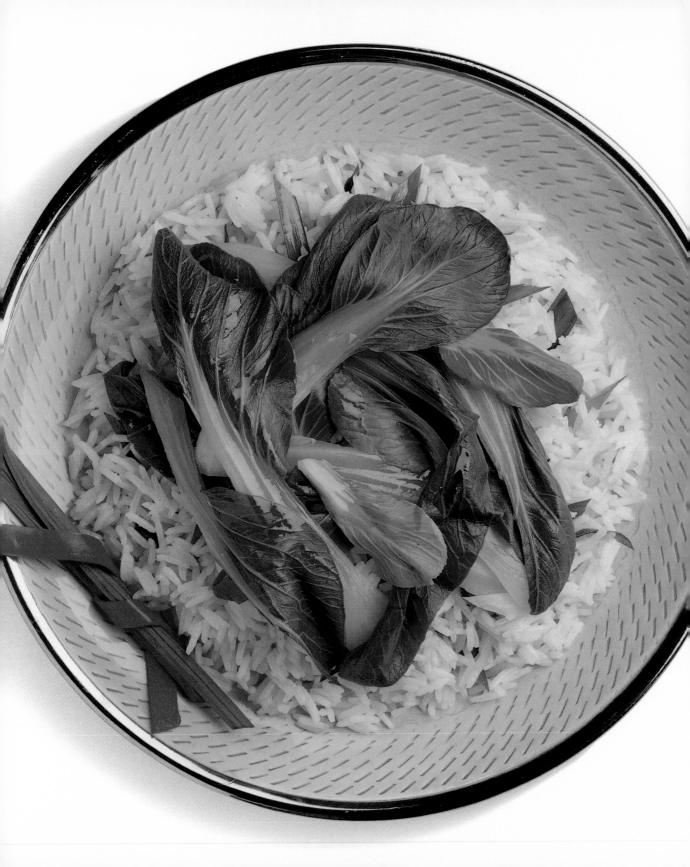

Asia's popular fried rice becomes a healthy main dish by eliminating the egg and reducing the oil. Bok choy is a delicately flavored cabbage variety with dark green leaves and crisp white stalks. Napa cabbage may be substituted and other vegetables added.

Stir-fried Rice

Serves 6

4 cups (32 fl oz/1 l) water
2 cups (14 oz/440 g) white rice
1 cup (8 fl oz/250 ml) Vegetable
 Stock or Chicken Stock
 (recipes on page 124)
1 star anise
1½ lb (750 g) bok choy, cut into
 wedges 3 inches (7.5 cm) wide

1 tablespoon peanut oil
2 oz (60 g) garlic chives or chives,
 cut into 1-inch (2.5-cm) lengths
1 tablespoon low-sodium soy sauce
1 tablespoon rice wine vinegar
½ teaspoon Flavored Sesame Oil
 (recipe on page 127)

1. In a medium saucepan over high heat bring the water to a boil. Add the rice, cover, reduce the heat to low and cook until the rice is fluffy, about 18 minutes.
2. In a large saucepan, combine the Vegetable or Chicken Stock, star anise and bok choy. Cover and bring to a boil over high heat. Reduce the heat to medium and simmer, covered, just long enough to soften the bok choy, about 5 minutes. Turn off the heat and discard the star anise. Re-cover and set aside.
3. In a wok or large frying pan over medium-low heat, warm the peanut oil. When the oil is hot, add the chives and cook, tossing and stirring, until the chives turn bright green, 20 seconds. Add the soy sauce and rice and toss just until the rice becomes crispy, about 2 minutes.
4. To serve, spoon the rice onto individual plates. Using a slotted spoon, lift out the bok choy from the stock and place on top of the rice. Sprinkle with the rice wine vinegar and Flavored Sesame Oil.

*Nutritional Analysis
Per Serving:*

**CALORIES 269
(KILOJOULES 1,129)
PROTEIN 7 G
CARBOHYDRATES 53 G
TOTAL FAT 3 G
SATURATED FAT 1 G
CHOLESTEROL 0 MG
SODIUM 157 MG
DIETARY FIBER 1 G**

Though wheat berries take a while to cook, their chewy texture and nutty flavor are well worth the trouble. They are rich in carbohydrates, protein, B vitamins, fiber and iron. The mixture also makes an excellent stuffing for roast poultry.

Wheat Berry & Rice Melange

Serves 6

1 cup (8 oz/250 g) wheat berries
5 cups (40 fl oz/1.25 l) water
¼ teaspoon sea salt
grated zest of 1 orange
1 cup (7 oz/220 g) fragrant rice
½ cup (4 fl oz/125 ml) Citrus
  Marinade made from lime juice
  and tequila *(recipe on page 127)*
  or fresh orange juice

¼ cup (2 fl oz/60 ml) walnut, peanut
  or olive oil
½ cup (3 oz/90 g) grated, peeled
  jicama or drained canned water chestnuts
½ cup (2 oz/60 g) pitted dried cherries,
  soaked in warm water to cover, plumped
  for 5 minutes and drained
1 navel orange, peeled, white pith removed
  and chopped
¼ cup (⅓ oz/10 g) chopped fresh mint

Nutritional Analysis Per Serving:

**Calories 343
(Kilojoules 1,441)
Protein 7 g
Carbohydrates 57 g
Total Fat 10 g
Saturated Fat 1 g
Cholesterol 0 mg
Sodium 66 mg
Dietary Fiber 1 g**

1. In a large saucepan, combine the wheat berries, 3 cups (24 fl oz/750 ml) of the water, the sea salt and half of the orange zest. Bring to a boil over high heat, reduce the heat to low, cover and simmer for 45 minutes.
2. Uncover and stir in the rice and the remaining 2 cups (16 fl oz/500 ml) water. Re-cover and continue to simmer over low heat for 20 minutes longer. Test at this point to see if the grains are tender and the liquid is absorbed; if not, re-cover and simmer for a few minutes longer. Remove from the heat and let stand, covered, for 5 minutes.
3. Fluff the grains with a fork, then spoon them into a large shallow bowl. Add the Citrus Marinade and toss to coat evenly. Let stand for 5 minutes to soak up the mixture. Then add the walnut oil and the remaining orange zest and toss again to mix well. Gently stir in the jicama or water chestnuts and cherries. Let the mixture cool thoroughly.
4. To serve, toss in the chopped orange and sprinkle with mint.

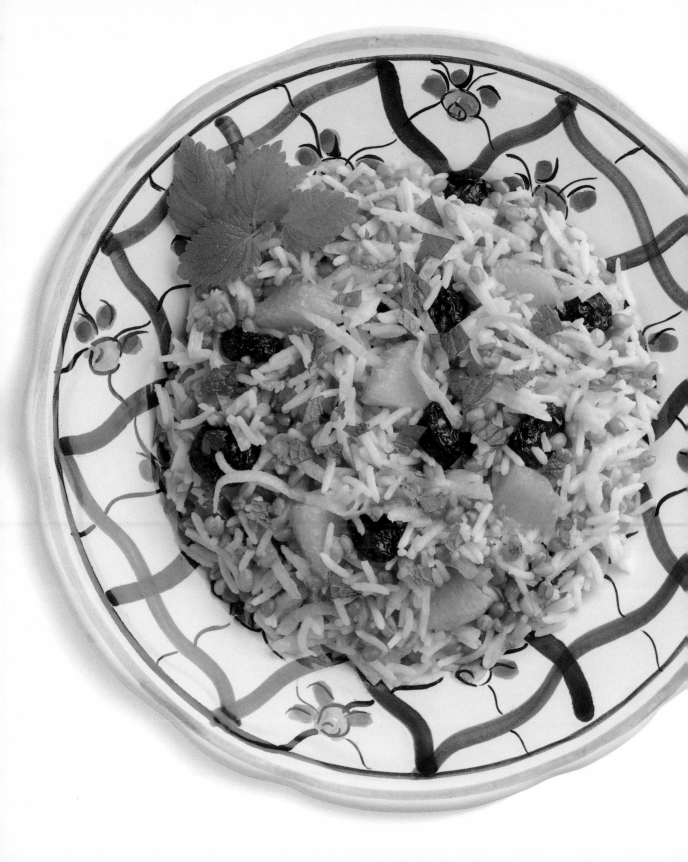

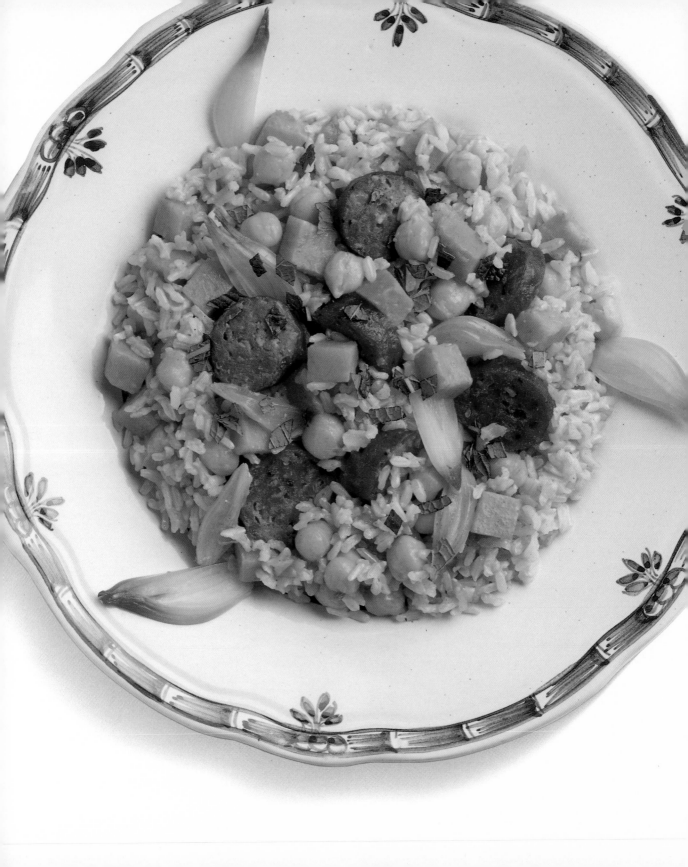

India's aromatic rice becomes a filling main course when cooked with chick-peas, sweet potatoes and a little meat. Orange-fleshed sweet potatoes are an excellent source of vitamin A and minerals. Leave out the meat for a lower-fat, vegetarian version.

BASMATI RICE & SAUSAGE PILAF

Serves 6

10 shallots

1 large or 2 medium sweet potatoes, peeled and cut into ½-inch (12-mm) dice

1 teaspoon olive oil

1½ lb (750 g) lamb or mild pork sausages

1 can (16 oz/500 g) chick-peas (garbanzo beans), drained

2 cups (14 oz/440 g) white or brown basmati rice

1 teaspoon ground cardamom

½ teaspoon ground cumin

4 cups (32 fl oz/1 l) Vegetable Stock or Chicken Stock *(recipes on page 124)* or water

½ teaspoon sea salt, optional

3 tablespoons fresh mint leaves, roughly chopped

1. Preheat an oven to 350°F (180°C).

2. Break apart the shallots into individual cloves but do not peel. Place in a shallow baking dish with the sweet potatoes. Drizzle with the olive oil.

3. Roast until the shallots are fragrant and soft when pierced, about 20 minutes. Let the vegetables cool slightly, then remove and discard the peels from the shallots. Leave the oven on.

4. While the vegetables cook, prick the sausages in a few places to allow the fat to drain off during cooking. Cook in a dry frying pan over medium heat, turning occasionally, until cooked through, about 15 minutes. Cut into slices ½ inch (12 mm) thick.

5. In a large, heavy ovenproof dish, combine the chick-peas, rice, cardamom, cumin, Vegetable or Chicken Stock or water, salt, if using, shallots, sweet potatoes and sausage. Stir to mix well. Cover and bake until the rice is tender, the liquid has been absorbed and holes appear in the surface of the rice, about 20 minutes.

6. To serve, sprinkle the mint over the top before scooping onto individual plates.

Nutritional Analysis Per Serving:

CALORIES 651
(KILOJOULES 2,736)
PROTEIN 29 G
CARBOHYDRATES 71 G
TOTAL FAT 30 G
SATURATED FAT 12 G
CHOLESTEROL 83 MG
SODIUM 193 MG
DIETARY FIBER 4 G

Red (or pink) lentils cook more quickly than the more common brown variety, speeding the preparation time in this adaptation of a North Indian vegetarian dish. The combination of lentils and rice provides a complete protein.

Lentils, Jasmine Rice & Vegetable Stir-fry

Serves 6

1 cup (7 oz/220 g) red lentils

2 cups (14 oz/440 g) basmati or jasmine rice

6 cups (48 fl oz/1.5 l) water

2 tablespoons plus 1 teaspoon olive oil

1 large yellow onion, finely diced

1 teaspoon ground coriander

1 cinnamon stick, about 4 inches (10 cm) long

4 green whole cardamom pods

2 bay leaves

3 whole cloves

⅛ teaspoon sea salt

1 tablespoon Roast Garlic Sauce *(recipe on page 126)* or 1 garlic clove, peeled and minced and mixed with 2 teaspoons white wine vinegar

1 teaspoon cumin seeds

2 red or green bell peppers (capsicums), seeded, deribbed and cut into long, narrow strips

1 zucchini (courgette), thinly sliced whole cilantro leaves

2 teaspoons Flavored Sesame Oil *(recipe on page 127)*

Nutritional Analysis Per Serving:

Calories 408

(Kilojoules 1,714)

Protein 17 g

Carbohydrates 73 g

Total Fat 9 g

Saturated Fat 1 g

Cholesterol 0 mg

Sodium 65 mg

Dietary Fiber 5 g

1. In a large bowl, combine the lentils and rice. Add the water. Let stand for 20 minutes. Drain, reserving the water.

2. In a large, heavy saucepan over medium heat, warm the 2 tablespoons olive oil. Add the onion and sauté, stirring, until golden and fragrant, 5–8 minutes. Push the onion to one side of the pan. Add the coriander, cinnamon stick, cardamom pods, bay leaves and cloves and heat, stirring, until the spices are lightly toasted, 20–30 seconds.

3. Stir in the drained rice and lentils and the salt. Add the reserved water, cover and cook over medium-low heat until the rice and lentils are done, about 20 minutes. The dish is ready when the water has been absorbed, the rice and lentils are tender and the surface of the rice is covered with small holes. Remove from the heat and let stand, covered, 5–10 minutes, to allow the starch in the grains to settle. Remove and discard the whole spices.

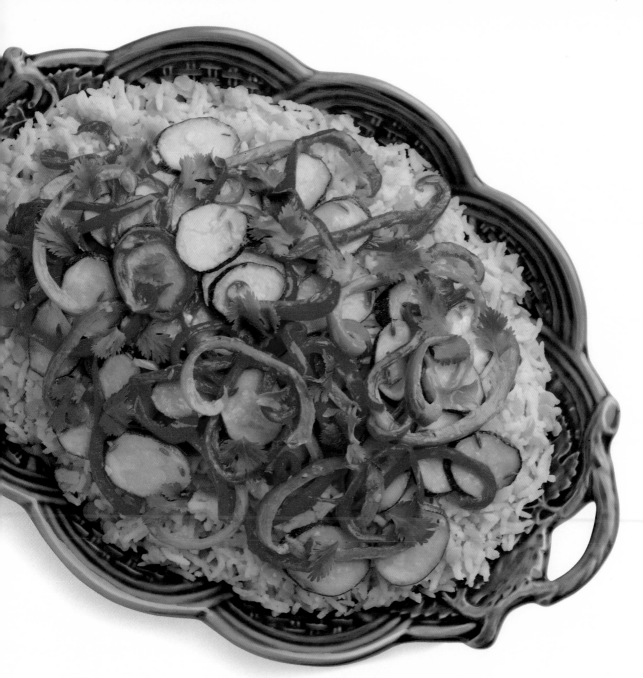

4. Meanwhile, in a frying pan over medium heat, warm the remaining 1 teaspoon olive oil. Add the Garlic Sauce. When the sauce is hot, add the cumin seeds, bell peppers and zucchini. Stir and toss until the vegetables are tender-crisp, 4–5 minutes.

5. To serve, spoon the rice mixture onto a large warmed serving platter. Top with the stir-fried vegetables. Sprinkle with the cilantro and drizzle with the Flavored Sesame Oil.

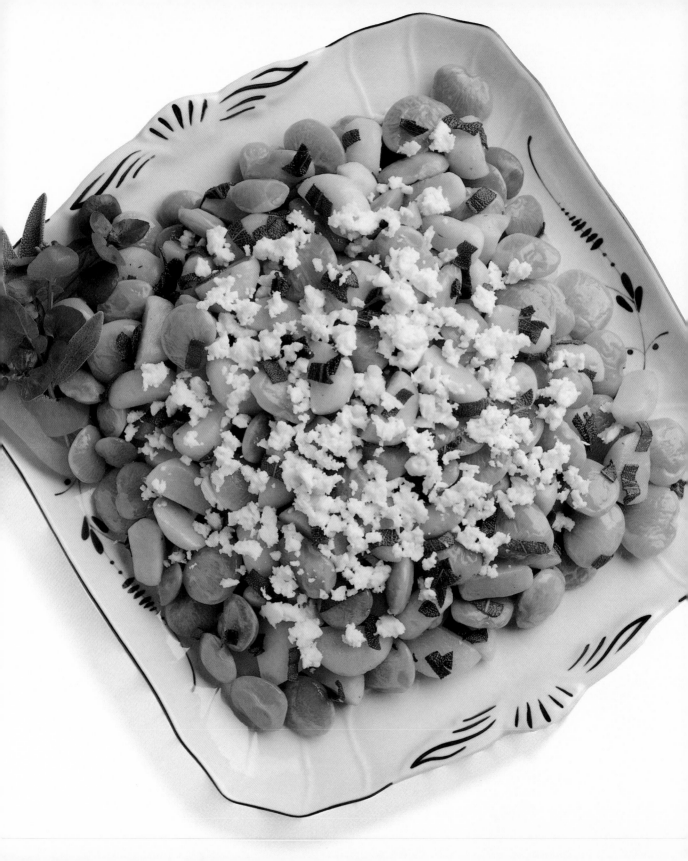

Both lima beans and water chestnuts provide a wealth of complex carbohydrates, and lima beans are also a good source of protein. Crumbled feta cheese adds extra zest to the mixture; be sure to rinse it first to remove excess salt.

LIMA BEAN & WATER CHESTNUT MEDLEY

Serves 6

2 tablespoons unsalted butter
16 oz (500 g) canned water chestnuts, drained and halved
1 lb (500 g) shelled fresh baby lima
  beans or frozen baby lima beans,
  thawed

¼ cup (¼ oz/8 g) fresh sage leaves,
  roughly chopped
2 oz (60 g) feta cheese, crumbled
  and rinsed to remove excess salt

1. In a frying pan over medium heat, melt the butter. Add the water chestnuts and sauté until softened, about 5 minutes.
2. Add the lima beans and sage and sauté until the lima beans are bright green, about 5 minutes longer.
3. To serve, transfer to a serving dish and top with the feta cheese.

Nutritional Analysis Per Serving:

CALORIES 198
(KILOJOULES 830)
PROTEIN 8 G
CARBOHYDRATES 29 G
TOTAL FAT 6 G
SATURATED FAT 4 G
CHOLESTEROL 19 MG
SODIUM 151 MG
DIETARY FIBER 0 G

Fresh white peas taste far creamier than their dry counterparts, making for a satisfying main dish high in complex carbohydrates. The range of choices is endless, from elegant little White Acres to black-eyed or crowder peas to large lima beans.

White Peas & Tomato Sauce Parmigiano

Serves 6

1½ lb (750 g) shelled white peas
6 cups (48 fl oz/1.5 l) Vegetable
  Stock *(recipe on page 124)* or water
½ cup (4 fl oz/125 ml) Quick
  Tomato Sauce *(recipe on page 126)*
½ teaspoon sea salt

¼ teaspoon freshly ground pepper
2 large ripe tomatoes, cut into chunks
3 tablespoons fresh basil leaves,
  roughly chopped
1 oz (30 g) Parmesan cheese, cut into
  thick slices

1. In a large saucepan over high heat, combine the peas, Vegetable Stock or water and Quick Tomato Sauce. When the mixture begins to boil, reduce the heat to medium-low, cover and simmer for 15 minutes.

2. Uncover, add the salt and pepper and simmer to reduce and thicken the broth, 5–10 minutes longer. As they cook, the peas will start to burst, releasing their starch into the flavorful liquid.

3. To serve, spoon the peas into deep individual bowls. Top with the tomatoes, basil and cheese.

Nutritional Analysis Per Serving:

CALORIES 198
(KILOJOULES 834)
PROTEIN 11 G
CARBOHYDRATES 35 G
TOTAL FAT 2 G
SATURATED FAT 0 G
CHOLESTEROL 4 MG
SODIUM 231 MG
DIETARY FIBER 1 G

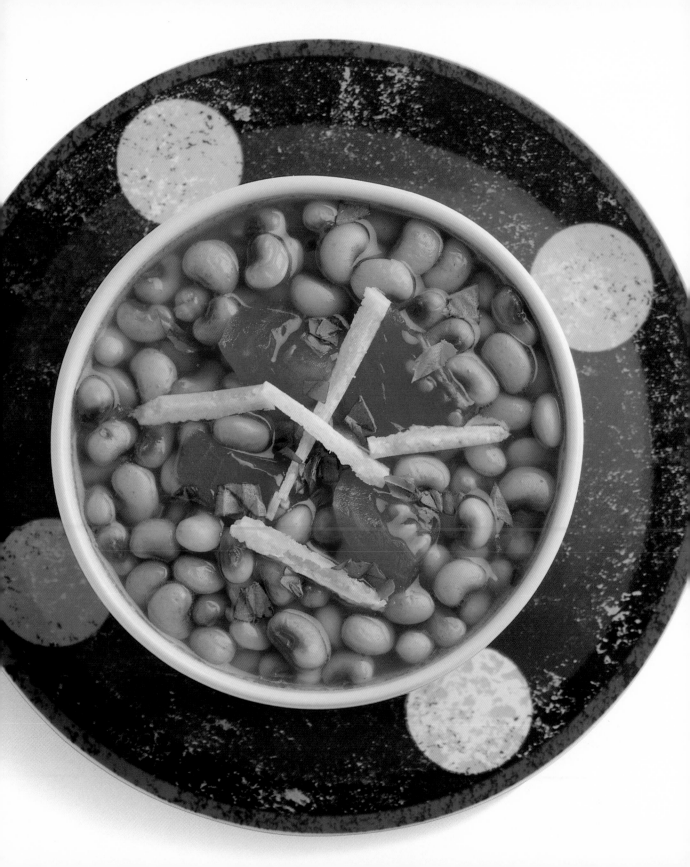

Adding a little chorizo sausage elevates the classic duo of beans and rice to hearty main dish status, without diminishing its healthfulness. Be sure to cook the peppers and onions for the full time given; the longer they cook, the deeper their flavors.

BLACK BEANS & YELLOW RICE

Serves 6

¼ lb (125 g) chorizo, diced
1 large white onion, chopped
1 large green bell pepper (capsicum),
  seeded, deribbed and diced
1 fresh jalapeño pepper, seeded
  and minced
1 teaspoon ground cumin
2 bay leaves
2 cans (16 oz/500 g each) black
  beans, drained and rinsed
3 cups (24 fl oz/750 ml) Vegetable
  Stock *(recipe on page 124)* or water

1 tablespoon cider vinegar
1 cup (7 oz/220 g) white rice
1 teaspoon ground turmeric
¼ teaspoon sea salt
2 tablespoons Roast Garlic Sauce
  (recipe on page 126) or 2 garlic cloves,
  peeled and minced and mixed with
  1 tablespoon white wine vinegar
½ cup (4 oz/125 g) lowfat plain yogurt
¼ cup (¼ oz/ 8 g) fresh cilantro (fresh
  coriander) leaves, roughly chopped

1. In a deep frying pan or heavy saucepan over medium heat, fry the chorizo, stirring, until it renders its fat and becomes crispy, about 8 minutes. Stir in the onion and bell pepper, reduce the heat to medium–low and cook, stirring, until the vegetables are very tender and fragrant, 10–15 minutes.

2. Stir in the jalapeño pepper, cumin, bay leaves, black beans and 1 cup (8 fl oz/250 ml) of the Vegetable Stock or water and bring to a simmer. Cook, uncovered, for 10 minutes. Remove and discard the bay leaves. Drizzle the cider vinegar over the beans, cover and keep warm until serving.

3. While the beans are simmering, in a saucepan, bring the remaining 2 cups (16 fl oz/500 ml) Vegetable Stock to a boil. Stir in the rice, turmeric and salt, cover, reduce the heat to low and simmer until the rice is tender and the liquid is absorbed, 18–20 minutes.

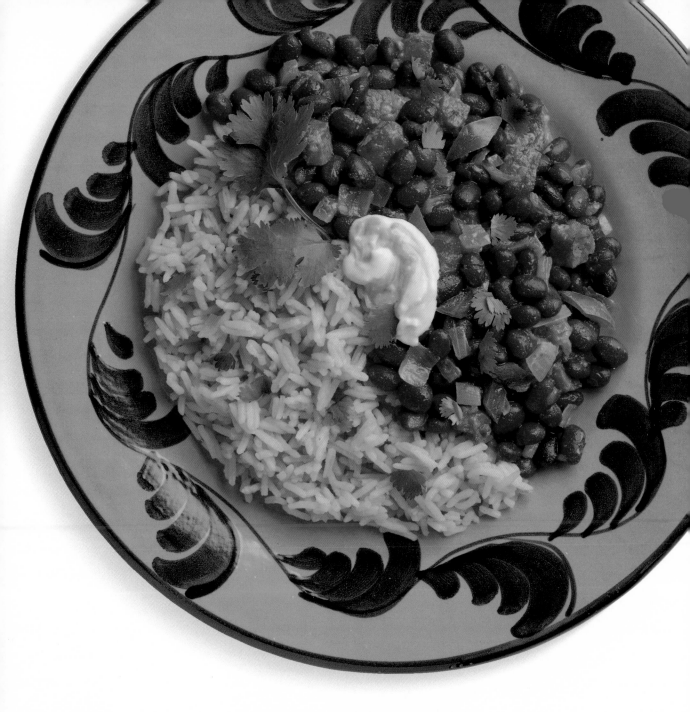

4. In a small bowl, stir together the Garlic Sauce and yogurt only until it looks marbleized; do not completely blend it. Set aside.
5. To serve, spoon the rice onto individual plates and top with the beans. Spoon the garlic-yogurt mixture over beans and sprinkle with the cilantro.

BASIC TERMS & TECHNIQUES

The following entries provide a reference source for this volume, offering definitions of essential or unusual ingredients and explanations of fundamental cooking techniques.

BEANS

Beans provide an important source of protein, fiber and complex carbohydrates in healthy main dishes; they are also good sources of essential B vitamins and minerals. Before use, dried beans should be carefully picked over to remove any impurities such as small stones or fibers or any discolored or misshapen beans. Presoak beans in cold water to cover for a few hours to rehydrate them, shorten their cooking time and improve their digestibility. Rinse canned beans well with cold water to flush out excess sodium.

Dozens of different kinds of beans are used in cuisines worldwide; some of the more common varieties used in this volume include:

BABY LIMA BEANS Small variety of flat, white, kidney-shaped beans with a mild flavor and soft texture. Larger dried lima beans may be substituted. Lima beans are also available fresh in season, as well as frozen.

BLACK BEANS Earthy-tasting, mealy-textured beans, relatively small in size and with deep black skins. Also called turtle beans.

BLACK-EYED PEAS Small, bean-shaped peas, rich in flavor and with a distinctive black dot on their otherwise ivory skins.

CANNELLINI BEANS Italian variety of small, white, thin-skinned, oval beans. Great Northern or white (navy) beans may be substituted.

CHICK-PEAS Round, tan-colored member of the pea family, with a slightly crunchy texture and nut-like flavor. Also known as garbanzo or ceci beans.

WHITE (NAVY) BEANS Small, white, thin-skinned, oval beans. Also known as Boston beans. Great Northern beans may be substituted.

BUTTER

For the recipes in this book, unsalted butter is preferred. Lacking salt, it allows the cook greater leeway in seasoning recipes to taste or dietary needs.

CHEESES

Although most cheeses are high in fat and therefore largely excluded in large quantities from health-conscious diets, just a little cheese can go a long way to add hints of flavor and richness to healthy main dishes. Cheese is also an excellent source of calcium.

These highly flavored cheeses are a good choice when used sparingly in a healthy diet:

FETA White, salty, sharp-tasting cheese made from sheep's or goat's milk, with a crumbly, creamy-to-dry consistency.

PARMESAN Hard, thick-crusted Italian cow's milk cheese, partially skimmed, with a sharp, salty, full flavor resulting from 1½–2 years of aging. For best flavor, buy in block form, to grate fresh as needed, rather than already grated.

PECORINO Italian sheep's milk cheese, sold either fresh or aged. Two of its most popular aged forms are pecorino romano and pecorino sardo; the latter cheese is tangier than the former.

SAPSAGO Hard, pungent, light-green-colored grating cheese from Switzerland, with a fat content of less than 10 percent.

CITRUS FRUITS

The thin, brightly colored, outermost layer of a citrus fruit's peel, the zest contains most of its aromatic essential oils—a lively source of flavor. The flesh of citrus fruit contains remarkable amounts of vitamin C.

To Section Citrus Fruit: Using a small, sharp knife, cut a thick slice off the bottom and top of the citrus fruits, exposing the fruit beneath the peel. Then, steadying the fruit on a work surface, thickly slice off the peel in strips, cutting off the white pith with it. Hold the peeled fruit in one hand over a bowl to catch the juices. Using the same knife, carefully cut on each side of the membrane to free each section, letting the sections drop into the bowl as they are cut.

To Zest Citrus Fruit: Using a zester or a fine hand-held shredder, draw its sharp-edged holes across the fruit's skin to remove the zest in thin strips. Alternatively, holding the edge of a paring knife or vegetable peeler away from you and almost parallel to the skin, carefully cut off the zest in thin strips, taking care not to remove any white pith with it.

DAIRY PRODUCTS

The rich, mild flavor of milk and milk products can be incorporated into main dishes with little or none of the fat present in whole milk, which contains 3.3 percent fluid fat and thus derives almost half of its calories from fat. Lowfat milk with 2 percent fluid fat, by contrast, gets only 35 percent of its calories from fat; lowfat milk with 1 percent fluid fat has only 23 percent of calories from fat; and nonfat milk typically derives only 5 percent of calories from fat. Lowfat buttermilk, although it has a rich, tangy flavor

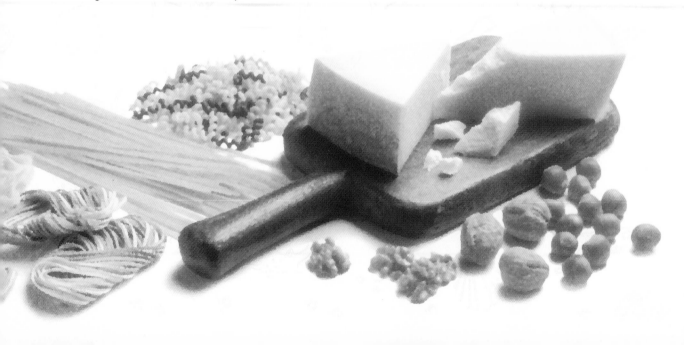

and thick, creamy texture, has just 1.5 percent fluid fat and derives 20 percent of calories from fat. Similar percentages also apply to yogurt, a substitute for sour cream. Canned evaporated skim milk is equally low in fat, and, like buttermilk, may be used to make rich, smooth sauces. All dairy products are a primary source of calcium and vitamins A and D.

GARLIC

This pungent bulb is popular worldwide in both raw and cooked form. Generally used unpeeled and minced, raw garlic is quite pungent, but cooking renders it mild to almost sweet. Use garlic in a healthy diet to replace flavor lost when fat and sodium are reduced and as a thickening agent for sauces. Choose plump, firm whole heads. Purchase only what you will use in 1–2 weeks, as garlic can shrivel and loose flavor with prolonged storage. Store whole heads in a cool, dark place; individual cloves dry out very quickly. Store minced garlic in the refrigerator.

To Peel a Garlic Clove: Place on a work surface and cover with the side of a large chef's knife. Press down firmly but carefully on the side of the knife to crush the clove slightly; the dry skin will then slip off easily.

HERBS

Use versatile and colorful culinary herbs for garnishing, for mixing into butters, for flavoring oils and vinegars and as an alternative to salt for seasoning recipes. Keep fresh herbs in water—as you do cut flowers—awaiting use. They will last up to 1 week, if trimmed daily, decorating and scenting your kitchen before flavoring and garnishing your food. Store dried herbs in tightly covered containers in a cool, dark place and use within six months of purchase.

To Chop Fresh Herbs: Wash the herbs under cold running water and thoroughly shake dry. If the herb has leaves attached along woody stems, strip the leaves from the stems. Otherwise, hold the stems together, gather up the leaves into a tight, compact bunch and, using a chef's knife, carefully cut across the bunch to chop the leaves coarsely. Discard the stems.

To Crush Dried Herbs: If using dried herbs, it is best to crush them first in the palm of the hand to release their flavor. Or warm them in a frying pan and crush using a mortar and pestle.

MISO

A thick, rich-tasting paste fermented from cooked soybeans, wheat or rice, and salt, used as a seasoning in Japanese cooking. The two most common forms are the more robust red miso (or

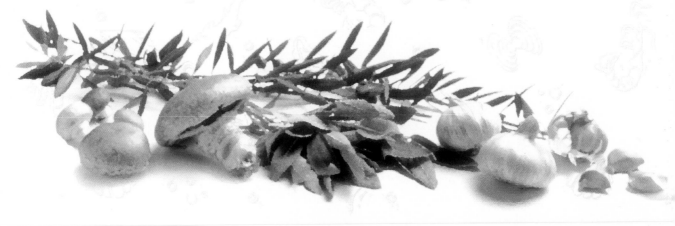

miso) and the milder white miso (shiro miso). Available in Japanese food shops and some well-stocked food markets.

MUSHROOMS

With their meaty textures and rich, earthy flavors, mushrooms enrich many main dishes. Cultivated white and brown mushrooms are widely available in food markets and green grocers; in their smallest form, with their caps still closed, they are often descriptively called button mushrooms. Cremini, similar in shape to cultivated mushrooms, are generally somewhat larger, mottled brown in color and have a meatier flavor and texture. Shiitakes, meaty-flavored Asian mushrooms, have flat, dark brown caps usually 2–3 inches (5–7.5 cm) in diameter and are available fresh with increasing frequency, particularly in Asian food shops. They are also sold dried, requiring soaking in warm water to cover for approximately 20 minutes before use. Portobello mushrooms have wide, flat, deep-brown caps with a rich, mildly meaty flavor and a silken texture; growing in popularity, they are available in well-stocked food stores. White, gray or pinkish oyster mushrooms, another popular Asian variety with lily-shaped caps, are sold fresh in Asian markets and well-stocked food stores.

NONSTICK COOKING SPRAY

An aerosol mixture of oil, lecithin (a soybean extract used as an emulsifier), sometimes grain alcohol and a harmless propellant, nonstick cooking spray allows a fine mist of oil to be applied to a cooking surface or food, thus preventing food from sticking and enabling you to sauté, fry or grill with little added fat.

NUTS

Although nuts are high in fat and should therefore be avoided in large quantities in a health-conscious diet, they contribute their characteristic flavor and texture, as well as many hard-to-get vitamins and minerals.

OILS

Oils not only provide a medium in which foods may be browned without sticking, but also subtly enhance the flavor of recipes in which they are used. Though oil is nothing more than a vegetable fat that is liquid at room temperature, and therefore derives 100 percent of its calories from fat, a relatively small amount of oil can nonetheless aid cooking and add distinctive flavor. Oils are also an excellent source of vitamin E and play an essential role in transporting the fat-soluble vitamins in our diet. Vegetable oils contain no cholesterol. Store all oils in tightly covered containers in a cool, dark place.

OLIVE OIL With its rich flavor and range of uses, olive oil deserves its reputation as the queen of culinary oils. Medical studies show that monounsaturated fat, which is found in olive oil, may reduce the risk of heart disease, cancer and diabetes. Olive oils are identified by their acidity. Extra-virgin olive oil is the finest. Its low acidity makes it smooth on the palate when used in uncooked dishes or added to hot dishes at the end of cooking. Both virgin and pure olive oil have a slightly higher acidity level and are fine for cooked dishes.

PEANUT OIL Pale gold peanut oil has a subtle hint of the peanut's richness. Its high flash point makes it a good choice for stir frying.

SESAME OIL Rich, flavorful and aromatic sesame oil is pressed from sesame seeds. Sesame oils from China and Japan are made with toasted sesame seeds, resulting in a dark, strong oil used as a flavoring ingredient; their low smoking temperature makes them unsuitable for using alone for cooking. Cold-pressed sesame oil, made from untoasted seeds, is lighter in color and taste and may be used for cooking.

VEGETABLE & SEED OILS Flavorless vegetable and seed oils such as safflower, corn and canola (rapeseed) are employed for their high cooking temperatures and bland flavor.

WALNUT OIL Popular in dressings and as a seasoning, walnut oil conveys the rich taste of the nuts from which it is pressed; seek out oil made from lightly toasted nuts, which has a full but not too assertive flavor.

PASTA

The growing popularity of pasta as a healthy staple rich in complex carbohydrates and proteins has resulted in an ever widening range of pasta choices available in food stores and specialty shops. Choose from both fresh and dried pastas, made with or without eggs, and plain or flavored with a variety of vividly colored seasonings.

To Cook Pasta: Use enough boiling water to let the pasta circulate freely; salting the water is not necessary. For 1 lb (500 g), you'll need about 5 qt (5 l) of water. Cooking time will depend on pasta shape, size and dryness, with fresh pasta generally taking 1-3 minutes and dried 3-15 minutes. Check suggested times on packaging and test for doneness by removing a piece, letting it cool briefly and then biting into it.

PEPPERS

The widely varied pepper family ranges in form and taste from large, mild bell peppers (capsicums) to tiny, spicy-hot chilies.

Fresh, sweet-fleshed bell peppers are most common in the unripe green form, although ripened red or yellow varieties are also available. All bell peppers (capsicums) are a good source of vitamin C.

Red, ripe chilies are sold fresh and dried. Fresh green chilies include the mild-to-hot, dark green poblano, which resembles a tapered, triangular bell pepper; the long, mild Anaheim, or New Mexican; and the small, fiery serrano and jalapeño. When handling chilies, wear kitchen gloves to prevent any cuts or abrasions on your hands from contacting the peppers' volatile oils and take special care not to touch your eyes or other sensitive areas.

To Seed Raw Peppers: Cut the pepper in half lengthwise with a sharp knife. Pull out the stem section from each half, along with the cluster of seeds attached to it.

Remove any remaining seeds, along with any thin white membranes, or ribs, to which they are attached.

RICE

Among the many varieties of rice grown, milled and cooked around the world, the most popular are long-grain white rices, whose slender grains steam to a light, fluffy consistency. Seek out some of the more fragrant, flavorful varieties such as basmati and jasmine rice. Carefully follow cooking instructions on the package.

To Cook Rice: Allow 2 cups of water for every cup of uncooked rice. Bring the water to a boil and add the rice; when the water returns to a boil, reduce the heat to very low, cover and cook, without uncovering, until all the water has been absorbed and the rice is tender—usually about 20 minutes for long-grain white rice. Unpolished brown rice retains more fiber and nutrients, including B vitamins, than white rice. Because it still has the bran, brown rice needs to be cooked slightly longer and with more water than white rice.

SOY SAUCE

A very popular Asian seasoning and condiment, soy sauce is made from soybeans, wheat, salt and water. Chinese brands tend to be markedly saltier than Japanese. If you wish to cut your sodium intake, seek out one of the many low-sodium soy sauces now available commercially, which may have as much as 40 percent less salt than ordinary soy sauces.

STOCK

This flavorful liquid, used as the primary cooking liquid or moistening and flavoring agent in many recipes, is derived from slowly simmering chicken, meat, fish or vegetables in water, along with herbs and aromatic vegetables. Stock may be made fairly easily at home and can be frozen for future use *(recipes on page 124)*. Many good-quality canned stocks or broths, in regular or concentrated form, are also available; they tend to be saltier than homemade stock, however, so recipes in which they are used should be carefully tasted for seasoning.

TOFU

Also known as bean curd, this soft, custardlike curd is made from the milky liquid extracted from fresh soybeans, caused to solidify by a coagulating agent. Popular throughout Asia, fresh bean curd, packaged in water or in ultraheat-sterilized vacuum packs, is widely available in Asian markets as well as in some food stores, and is available in soft, medium-soft and firm varieties. Before use, drain tofu well and let it sit for about 15 minutes on several layers of paper towels to absorb excess moisture; follow recipe preparation instructions precisely to get the desired consistency. Tofu is a good source of non-meat protein and, depending on processing, can be rich in calcium.

TOMATOES

During the summer, when tomatoes are in season, use the best sun-ripened tomatoes you can find; at other times of year, plum tomatoes, sometimes called Roma or egg tomatoes, are likely to have the best flavor and texture. Small cherry tomatoes, barely bigger than the fruit after which they are descriptively named, also have a pronounced tomato flavor.

Seek out fresh tomatoes with a deep red color that are firm to the touch and store them in a cool, dark place. Refrigeration causes them to break down. Use within a few days of purchase. All tomatoes are a good source of vitamin C.

When good fresh tomatoes are not available, canned whole plum tomatoes can be used for cooking purposes. If you are following a low-sodium diet, seek out a brand that packages them without added salt.

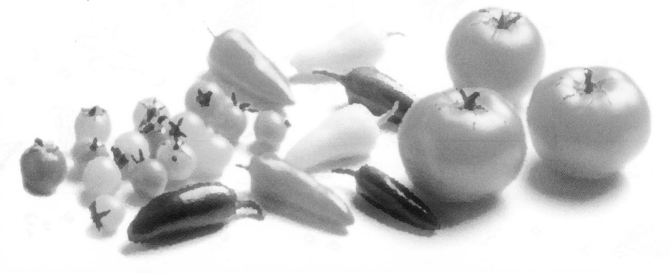

Basic recipes

Designed to be made ahead, stored and added to many of the dishes throughout this volume, these recipes provide fresh, preservative-free alternatives to similar commercial products.

Chicken Stock

Try making this stock with a roaster or stewing hen, which require longer simmering than a fryer but produce very flavorful results.

Makes about 1 qt (1 l)

2–3 lb (1–1.5 kg) mixed chicken pieces
  including backs and necks
1 large yellow onion, diced
1 large turnip or rutabaga, peeled and diced
½ teaspoon salt
½ teaspoon freshly ground pepper
2 bay leaves

1. Put the chicken pieces in a large stockpot and add water to cover. Bring to a boil, reduce the heat to medium-low and simmer, skimming off any surface scum.
2. When scum no longer forms on the surface, add the onion, turnip, salt, pepper and bay leaves to the pot. Cover partially and simmer for 30 minutes to 2 hours. The timing will depend upon the type of chicken.
3. Strain the stock through a sieve into a shallow container. Discard the solids. Let cool, cover and refrigerate overnight.
4. The next day, spoon off the fat that has solidified on the surface and discard. Store in a tightly covered container in the refrigerator for up to 3 days or in the freezer for 2 months.

Per 1 Cup Serving: Calories 40 (Kilojoules 167), Protein 2 g, Carbohydrates 5 g, Total Fat 1 g, Saturated Fat 0 g, Cholesterol 0 mg, Sodium 324 mg, Dietary Fiber 1 g

Vegetable Stock

This full-flavored stock is ideal for moistening vegetarian recipes. Sea salt, a mixture of magnesium chloride and potassium chloride, adds a purer flavor than conventional table salt and has less sodium by weight.

Makes about 3 qt (3 l)

3 qt (3 l) water
1 large yellow onion, unpeeled and roughly
  chopped
1 leek, carefully washed and roughly cut in rounds
3 large carrots, unpeeled and sliced
1 turnip, roughly chopped
6 thick celery stalks with leaves, cut into 2-inch
  (5-cm) pieces
2 bay leaves
1½ cups (5 oz/130 g) mushroom stems
sea salt

1. In a large stockpot over high heat, bring the water to a boil. Reduce the heat to medium-low and add the onion, leek, carrots, turnip, celery, bay leaves, mushroom stems and salt to taste. Cover or partially cover; simmer for 30 minutes.
2. Strain the stock through a sieve into a shallow container. Discard the solids. Let cool, cover and refrigerate for up to 5 days or freeze for up to 2 months.

Per 1 Cup Serving: Calories 12 (Kilojoules 52), Protein 0 g, Carbohydrates 3 g, Total Fat 0 g, Saturated Fat 0 g, Cholesterol 0 mg, Sodium 12 mg, Dietary Fiber 1 g

SEASONED BREAD CRUMBS & CROUTONS

Both bread crumbs and croutons may be stored in a tightly covered container in the pantry for up to 1 week or in the freezer for up to 3 months.

Makes about 4 cups crumbs (16 oz / 500 g)

½ lb (250 g) slightly stale, good-quality French, Italian, rye or whole-wheat bread
1 tablespoon olive oil
2 tablespoons chopped fresh oregano, thyme, lemon thyme, sage, flat-leaf (Italian) parsley or basil leaves or a mixture of herbs

1. Preheat a broiler (griller).
2. To make bread crumbs, cut the bread into slices ½ inch (12 mm) thick and then break the slices into large pieces. Place on a baking sheet in a single layer and broil (grill) for 2 minutes, turning over after 1 minute. Transfer the toasted bread to a food processor fitted with the metal blade. Add the olive oil and herbs and process until finely ground, about 20 seconds.
3. To make croutons, cut the bread into ½ inch (12 mm) thick slices and then cut the slices into ½-inch (12-mm) cubes. Place in a large bowl. Add the olive oil and herbs and toss to coat the bread cubes evenly. Spread the bread cubes in a single layer on a baking sheet and place in the broiler. Broil (grill) until golden, for 2 minutes, turning over after 1 minute.
4. Let the crumbs or croutons cool completely before using or storing.

Seasoned Bread Crumbs Per ¼ Cup Serving: Calories 47 (Kilojoules 196), Protein 1 g, Carbohydrates 7 g, Total Fat 1 g, Saturated Fat 0 g, Cholesterol 0 mg, Sodium 86 mg, Dietary Fiber 0 g
Seasoned Croutons Per ¼ Cup Serving: Calories 34 (Kilojoules 143), Protein 1 g, Carbohydrates 5 g, Total Fat 1 g, Saturated Fat 0 g, Cholesterol 0 mg, Sodium 63 mg, Dietary Fiber 0 g

NUT CRUMBS

Makes about 1 cup (4 oz / 125 g)

1 cup (4–5 oz / 125–155 g) shelled nuts

1. Preheat an oven to 300°F (150°C).
2. Place the nuts in a single layer on a baking sheet. Toast until golden and fragrant, 5–8 minutes. Let cool and chop coarsely.
3. Transfer the nuts to the work bowl of a food processor fitted with the metal blade. Process briefly using short pulses. Do not allow the nuts to turn to paste.
4. Let cool completely before using. To store, wrap tightly and freeze for up to 1 month.

Per 1 Tablespoon Serving, based on walnuts: Calories 51 (Kilojoules 215), Protein 1 g, Carbohydrates 1 g, Total Fat 5 g, Saturated Fat 0 g, Cholesterol 0 mg, Sodium 1 mg, Dietary Fiber 0 g

QUICK TOMATO SAUCE

*If good fresh tomatoes are unavailable,
substitute 2 cans (24 oz/750 g each) plum
tomatoes, without their juices.*

Makes about 8 cups (64 fl oz/2 l)

3 lb (1.5 kg) ripe plum (Roma) tomatoes
2 tablespoons olive oil
1 large white onion, thickly sliced
4 garlic cloves, smashed
2 tablespoons chopped fresh oregano leaves
  or 1 tablespoon dried oregano leaves
½ cup (½ oz/15 g) fresh flat-leaf (Italian)
  parsley, stems and leaves, left whole
1 tablespoon balsamic vinegar
1 teaspoon vodka

1. Fill a saucepan three-fourths full of water
and bring to a boil. Fill a large bowl half full
of cold water.
2. Cut a shallow cross in the blossom end of
each tomato. When the water boils, immerse the
tomatoes in it for 1 minute. Using a slotted
spoon, transfer the tomatoes to the cold water.
When cool enough to handle, using the tip
of a paring knife, pull off the peel and discard.
Coarsely chop the tomatoes.
3. In a large deep frying pan over medium heat,
warm the olive oil. Add the onion and sauté
slowly until fragrant and translucent, 5–10 minutes. Add the garlic, oregano, parsley, balsamic
vinegar and vodka and toss lightly to mix.
4. Stir in the tomatoes. Reduce the heat to
medium-low; cook the sauce, uncovered, stirring occasionally, until slightly thickened, about
10 minutes. Remove and discard the parsley.

*Per 1 Cup Serving: Calories 79 (Kilojoules 333),
Protein 2 g, Carbohydrates 11 g, Total Fat 4 g,
Saturated Fat 1 g, Cholesterol 0 mg, Sodium 18 mg,
Dietary Fiber 3 g*

ROAST GARLIC SAUCE

*While you can substitute peeled and minced fresh
garlic mixed with vinegar for this sauce, cooking
mellows the garlic flavor. Make this basic recipe
regularly and keep some stored in the refrigerator
to add flavor and texture to many dishes.*

Makes about 2 cups (16 fl oz/500 ml)

6 garlic heads in the husk (12 oz/375 g)
4 tablespoons (2 fl oz/60 ml) virgin olive oil
3 large fresh thyme sprigs or 1 teaspoon
  dried thyme
½ cup (4 fl oz/125 ml) white wine vinegar
2 tablespoons balsamic vinegar
freshly ground pepper

1. Preheat an oven to 300°F (150°C).
2. Pull open each garlic head. Drizzle an equal
amount of 1 tablespoon of the olive oil into
each head. Place the garlic and thyme in a small
baking pan and cover tightly with aluminum
foil. Roast until the garlic is soft when pierced
with a knife, about 45 minutes.
3. Using the back of a fork, press the garlic
pulp out of the husk. Pull the thyme leaves
from the stems and discard the stems.
4. Combine the remaining 3 tablespoons olive
oil and the cooled garlic and thyme in a bowl
and, using a fork, mash until smooth.
Alternatively, in a food processor fitted with the
metal blade, combine the olive oil, garlic and
thyme and process until smooth. Add the wine
vinegar, balsamic vinegar and pepper to taste
and stir or process until smooth. The sauce will
be creamy. Store in a tightly covered container
in the refrigerator for up to 1 week.

*Per 1 Tablespoon Serving: Calories 30 (Kilojoules 125),
Protein 1 g, Carbohydrates 3 g, Total Fat 2 g,
Saturated Fat 0 g, Cholesterol 0 mg, Sodium 2 mg,
Dietary Fiber 0 g*

CITRUS MARINADE

Appealingly tart, sweet and hot, this mixture may be used as a marinade or sauce, stirred into grain or pasta dishes or spooned over grilled fish or pork at the table.

Makes about 1 cup (8 fl oz/250 ml)

¾ cup (6 fl oz/180 ml) fresh orange juice or
   Key lime juice
1 teaspoon sugar
¼ teaspoon finely minced fresh green chili
   pepper
1 tablespoon snipped fresh cilantro (fresh
   coriander)
1 tablespoon light rum, if using orange juice
   or tequila, if using lime juice

1. In a large nonreactive bowl, combine the orange juice or lime juice, sugar, chili pepper and cilantro. Add the rum if using orange juice and the tequila if using lime juice. Let stand at room temperature for 30 minutes to 2 hours to develop the flavors.
2. Store in a tightly covered container in the refrigerator for up to 3 days.

Per 1 Teaspoon Serving: Calories 3 (Kilojoules 11), Protein 0 g, Carbohydrates 0 g, Total Fat 0 g, Saturated Fat 0 g, Cholesterol 0 mg, Sodium 0 mg, Dietary Fiber 0 g

FLAVORED SESAME OIL

Just a few drops of this fragrant oil add a burst of flavor to finished dishes. Use Asian toasted sesame oil, which has the most intense flavor.

Makes about 1 cup (8 fl oz/250 ml)

1 cup (8 fl oz/250 ml) Asian toasted sesame oil
zest of 2 tangerines or oranges, grated or cut
   into thin strips
1 teaspoon New Mexico or other ground dried
   pungent chili

1. In a small, heavy saucepan, combine the sesame oil, citrus zest and ground chili. Place over medium-low heat and cook until bubbles begin to break on the surface, 3–4 minutes.
2. Remove from the heat and let cool. Pour into a bottle, cap tightly and store in a cool, dark place indefinitely.

Per 1 Tablespoon Serving: Calories 121 (Kilojoules 510), Protein 0 g, Carbohydrates 0 g, Total Fat 14 g, Saturated Fat 2 g, Cholesterol 0 mg, Sodium 0 mg, Dietary Fiber 0 g

INDEX